Massage During Pregnancy

Bette L. Waters

RTP
Research Triangle Publishing

Published by
Research Triangle Publishing, Inc.
PO Box 1223
Fuquay-Varina, NC 27526

ISBN 1-884570-28-3

Library of Congress Catalog Card Number: 95-68164

Illustrations by
G&L Graphic Designs

Cover by
Kathy Holbrook

Edited by
Bonnie Tilson

Printed in the United States of America
10 9 8 7 6 5 4 3 2

TABLE OF CONTENTS

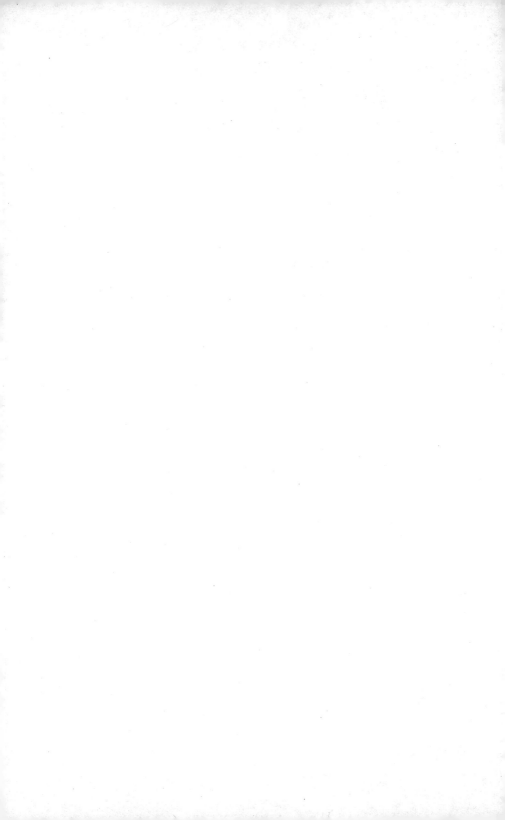

FOREWORD

I have been treating pregnant women for many years with various massage therapy techniques and often times the results have been amazing. One young mother, Kate (whose name has been changed for privacy's sake), comes to mind as an example of the power of precise massage therapy during pregnancy. Kate came to one of my neuromuscular training seminars with her mother specifically to show me her new infant. Kate's prior two pregnancies had resulted in cesarean section as she was told by her physician that her pelvis was too small to have a normal birth for the size babies that she carried. She had very long, difficult, and painful labors with her first two children. She was also advised that any future babies would need to be delivered by cesarean section.

This was Kate's third child and her mother, who was trained in Neuromuscular Therapy, St. John Method, treated her throughout the pregnancy. Kate's mother worked with her with specific Neuromuscular Therapy techniques such as pelvic stabilization and releasing muscles of the lower back, abdominal region, hips, and legs. These techniques helped to diminish the commonly seen increased lumbar lordosis and low back pain.

For Kate this dramatically decreased her discomfort during pregnancy, as well as during labor. She showed me her new infant and said with a big smile, "I delivered this child naturally. I did not need a C-section, my labor was only four hours long, and I had very little discomfort."

As I looked at the baby, I thought of the many children that I had seen with severe cranial distortions and other birth injuries, such as Klumpke's paralysis, a lower arm type of paralysis. I thought how unfortunate it is that so few people understand the tremendous role that massage therapy can play during pregnancy and the birthing process. I thought of how much future suffering for the child and mother could be prevented if people had adequate knowledge about massage and pregnancy.

I was delighted when Bette Waters asked me to write an introduction to *Massage During Pregnancy* because the vision of my company is to make massage therapy a viable health care option available to all people. Educating the public and health care professionals about the value of therapeutic massage is the first step.

The massage of pregnant women is shrouded with myths and superstitions. For instance, I have been told in my own state of Florida that I should not massage women who are pregnant. I have been told not only that I should not, but that I could not because it was against the law. When I looked for statutes to support this position, I found none—it was totally lawful.

First and foremost, the book separates superstition from fact. It provides the reader with an excellent understanding of the anatomy, physiology, and biochemical changes that take place during this wonderful gestation period when life is beginning to express itself.

Bette is to be commended for her extensive research in this very important area of massage. She discusses why certain positions are not advisable for the pregnant woman; the different stages of pregnancy including such changes as blood pressure, and the structure and functioning of the body; and the contraindications for massage during pregnancy.

Beyond all the facts—and there are many—is the sensitivity with which Bette approaches the experience of pregnancy. The lucid manner with which she presents the material gives the reader an empowering feeling that, "Yes, indeed, I can make a difference in the experience of pregnancy."

This is wonderful reading for the mother-to-be and her partner, as well as for the massage therapist who has pregnant clients. As I read the enlightening pages of this book, I felt as if I were actually participating in the birth experience. I wish that this book had been available before my three children were born. Although

I was present during the pregnancy and birth of each child, the entire process seemed like such a blur. At times I felt rather powerless even though I knew more than the average male about the process of birth.

Being male, I can only wonder what goes through the mind of a woman who is pregnant for the first time and begins to learn and experience all the discomforts of pregnancy. I have seen the fear about nausea, heartburn, sciatica, backaches, and headaches. What does it all mean? Not only will the reader learn what it all means, but more important, how to minimize it. Can you imagine how comforting it would be for the mother-to-be to learn and be able to anticipate the psychological adjustments that come with each trimester of pregnancy before she actually begins to experience these changes?

Another important area that *Massage During Pregnancy* addresses is the process of labor. Most of the fear that woman have about birth emanates from the stories they have heard about labor. Again, the information on the labor process is excellent for waylaying these fears.

I have observed for more than two decades the kind of precise post-traumatic soft tissue care people need in order to recover from and be pain free following traumatic events in their lives. Unfortunately, this precise type of soft tissue care is not widely known or used in our society.

For example, if you experience a traumatic event great enough to fracture a bone, you have a trauma great enough to do a lot of soft tissue damage. It is very common for people to experience pain coming from muscles, tendons, ligaments, and fascia long after the fracture has healed. This soft tissue pain usually increases over time. If proper soft tissue care is applied, this is not the case.

The same can be said about the trauma of childbirth. In the postpartum period and later, all too often I have heard women say things like, "I never had back pain before the birth of my child, but since that time, my back pain has steadily increased and now I am in constant pain."

Massage During Pregnancy does an excellent job of educating the health care professional as well as the patient about what emotional and physiological changes to expect and how to properly facilitate the healing process. Not only is postpartum care for the mother discussed, but also proper massage for the new baby. This process of infant massage is a wonderful assist in the bonding process, and has many health benefits for the child.

As with any information or therapeutic technique, massage for pregnancy is only as valuable as the love, experience, and scientific truth that goes with it. It will not take the reader long to become aware that the author possesses enough of all three of these qualities to make a significant contribution to any person's educational experience.

The knowledge and wisdom in this book will set new standards for the care of pregnant women in our society. I know the reader will enjoy the journey with Bette Waters into the beginning of life. Through the facilitation of human touch, this miracle of miracles, the birth of a child, can be elevated to new levels of joy and efficiency for both the parents and the child, and for the health care provider as well. This book will become required reading for all the patients that come to me for help during pregnancy.

This book is must reading for everyone involved in the healing arts, as well as those planning or expecting children. It is the kind of book that can change a society by making people more sensitive and humane. It is the kind of book that makes a difference.

Paul St. John, L.M.T.

PREFACE

How did we get involved in prenatal massage? I have been practicing nurse-midwifery in Central Florida for over eleven years and was a member of the first midwifery service to deliver women at Tampa General Hospital beginning in 1983. In 1988, Gerald (Jerry) Curwin, my husband, entered the Sarasota School of Massage as a student. He had made his living for years as an industrial engineer and later as the owner of a private trade school for landscaping and lawn maintenance education. Entry into massage school was the result of Jerry making a midlife career change in order to be a part of the entrepreneurial endeavor called New Image Wellness and Fitness Center—a business I had started for the benefit of women's health.

Returning home after class, many times, he would discuss with me his concerns about the contraindications for massaging pregnant women and the differing opinions of the faculty about whether you should or should not massage pregnant women. When he told me he was being taught that massage or stimulation of certain points of anatomy would cause labor, I was astounded. I said to him, "Do you know that if you could stimulate labor with massage, you could change obstetrical care?" Maybe I also alluded that he could become rich. He says the rich part is what inspired him.

Anyway, he chose massage of pregnant women as the subject for his school research paper. During work on his paper, he traveled to Tampa to the University of South Florida general library and its medical library to do a review of the literature. He found only two books and one foreign medical journal that mentioned massage.

A year later we began writing our research plan to study the effects of massage and its prevention of postdates in pregnancy. Our literature review was somewhat more successful when we began to look at the nursing literature and the non-traditional methods of birthing, e.g. home birth and birthing center movements. Many of these references appear in this book.

During this period of work, a vacation on the east coast of Florida took me to a massage school for stress reduction and relaxation necessary for a real vacation. During my massage I questioned one of the faculty members about massage of pregnant women. She told me there was a Florida State Law prohibiting massage therapists from providing massage to pregnant women. (I have been unable to find such a law in the statutes of Florida law.)

The anatomy and physiology education relating to muscles, nerves, and skeleton structure which Jerry received at his school was more intensive and in-depth than what I had been taught in my nursing education program. However, nothing about the male or female reproductive system was taught, nor was pregnancy discussed except as a contraindication for massage.

A video made and marketed to massage therapists and schools of massage teaching about massage for the pregnant woman made little reference to physiology of pregnancy. During the massage, the instructor on the video placed a woman who was 8 months pregnant in a supine position for massage. She made no reference to Supine Hypotensive Syndrome except to instruct her client to let her know if she felt dizzy while supine during the massage.

I share this information not to be critical, but to show what was being taught in some massage schools and what was available to the massage therapist seeking further information from the marketplace.

The evolution of these events convinced me that there was an enormous need for education based on scientific data directed toward the profession of massage and its role in pregnancy. And, indeed, if massage of certain anatomical points on the body could create labor, obstetrical care as we know it could be changed forever.

Based on our findings after many months and many hours in the libraries of the local university, Jerry and I began to market education seminars about massage in pregnancy. This material was approved for CEU's by the Florida State Board of Massage. The seminars offered regularly since October 1992 have been quite successful.

Today there is a window of opportunity for massage to become a part of routine obstetrical care. My mind boggles at the impact this event would have on the massage profession as well as pregnancy. Jerry and I will continue to produce the educational seminars on massage for the pregnant woman, but we feel we can reach many more therapists with this how-to book.

The infant massage movement began in this country in the 1980s and was designed to educate lay people, nurses, and childbirth educators about infant massage. It was not designed specifically to meet the needs and requirements of the massage profession. The infant massage techniques in this book are based on normal anatomy and physiology of the infant. Also, we have briefly included information about the scientific research done demonstrating the important positive effects of touch on the infant. Preparing your clients for the important advantages of learning to massage their children should be part of your service to the pregnant family.

ACKNOWLEDGMENTS

This book is the result of many people and events moving into and through my life over the past decade. One long-ago evening in Atlanta, Georgia, with Roberta Galliger, the idea for a "wellness center" was sparked while attending a seminar on women's health issues. Jayne Keller-Pace, RN, LMT provided hard work, sweat, and support to help turn the idea of a wellness center into walls and rooms.

Gerald Curwin, who brought love and appreciation into my life and launched me on the adventure of a lifetime, was always there as companion and best friend, offering advice, talk, and encouragement. I did not always take his advice, but I always listened because one idea out of a hundred could be brilliant. If you did not listen, you would miss the brilliance.

Special appreciation goes to my friend and mentor, Dr. Janet Askew Sipple. She has been a loving friend always, but also inspires me to do more than I imagine. Without her influence, the work on Ice Massage for Labor Pain would not have been done.

A special thank-you to Sue Morningstar, Nurse-Midwife, who served as editor and gave me great feedback and encouragement as each chapter evolved. Also, to Nancy Taschner, LMT and Laurete Beatriz Francescato, LMT who reviewed the chapters for clarity. I am indebted to Luis A. Acevedo-Rodriquez, M.D., FAAP, pediatrician, who reviewed the chapter on Infant Massage and gave me valuable suggestions.

A note of thanks to Nancy Schroeder, LMT in Texas where the book was finished. She not only reviewed for clarity the last versions of the hands-on and labor chapters, she also kept my stress level reduced with regular sessions on her massage table.

A special note of appreciation to Paul St. John, LMT for recognizing the value of this book. His encouragement kept me at the computer.

A note of appreciation to Gill and Lupe Rodriguez of G & L Graphic Designs, in Austin, Texas, whose talents are expressed in the art work.

I am especially indebted to the people who have come to the prenatal massage seminars and helped reinforce the need for the information offered in this book. I wish to express my heartfelt appreciation to each of you, named and unnamed, who participated in no small way in the evolution of this work.

Chapter One

THE ANATOMY AND PHYSIOLOGY OF PREGNANCY

The anatomical, physiological, and biochemical changes that take place in the woman during the 9-month period of gestation involve all systems of her body. These remarkable changes take place in response to physiological stimuli provided by the woman's reproductive system—ovaries, uterus, endocrine system—and the fetus.

The other amazing part of this process is that the pregnant woman returns almost completely to her prepregnancy state after delivery of her baby and her completion of lactation or nursing. The understanding of these changes and how they impact on the performance of massage on her body is one of the major goals of this book.

Keep in mind that the changes/adaptations examined are those that take place in the healthy female with a normal pregnancy. She is free from any disease processes caused by the pregnancy, and free from any disease existing before the pregnancy. I am not saying that the massage therapist should not be concerned with disease processes in the pregnant woman. However, it is not the role of the massage therapist to diagnose diseases. We will talk about risks involved with massaging pregnant women, and how to recognize and manage them.

With all the technology in medicine today, the United States is eighteenth in the world in prevention of infant death. A child born in Costa Rica has a better chance of surviving its first year than an infant born in this country. The major cause of this is premature birth. Medicine has determined the number one cause of premature birth is stress. You and I know the number one treatment for stress can be massage.

Thus, the pregnant woman has more of a need for routine massage because of the known association between increased stress and the onset of premature labor. However, there are some conditions, and some massage techniques and table positions that are contraindicated. These contraindications in the massage of pregnant women are discussed at length.

UTERUS

The uterus is truly a remarkable organ. The changes in this organ will have the greatest prenatal impact on modifying massage techniques and table positioning. The uterus has the capacity to increase rapidly in size during pregnancy and then return almost to its original size within a few weeks after delivery. The weight of the uterus will increase approximately 300 percent. Its size can increase up to 1,000 percent based on the size of the baby at birth.

In the nonpregnant woman the uterus is almost solid. It weighs 70 grams or approximately 3/4 pound and is pear shaped. It has a cavity that holds 10 milliliters, or 1/3 of an ounce. This cavity is not hollow, but folds in upon itself.

During the pregnancy the uterus grows into a thin-wall organ made of muscle large enough to hold more than 8 pounds of amniotic fluid, a pound and a half of placenta, plus the baby. At the end of the pregnancy it weighs approximately 1,100 grams or close to 2 and 1/2 pounds. This enlargement does not involve any increase in the number of muscle cells. The muscle cells themselves grow larger. There is an addition to the amount of surrounding collagen material. Other changes include an accumulation of fibrous tissue, particularly in the external muscle layer, and an increase in elastic material.

This network of muscle and fibrous tissue adds greatly to the strength of the uterine wall. And, of course, the uterus has to be strong in order to do the work of pushing the baby into the world at birth.

At the same time as the increase in muscle, fibrous, and collagen tissue, there is a great increase in the size and number of blood vessels and lymphatics. The veins that drain the placental site are transformed into large uterine sinuses. This is to provide for the exchange of food and oxygen from the mother to the fetus and waste products from the fetus to the mother. There is also an increase in the size of the uterine nerves. This rapid growth is due to an increase in growth hormones produced in the tissues of the wall of the pregnant uterus.

The uterus is a pelvic organ, resting atop the bladder. The lower portion of the uterus is called the cervix. The cervix is long and narrow and opens downward into the back of the vagina. (See Figure 1.) The uterus is supported by the round ligament, which attaches to the uterus near the fundus, or top of the uterus, and lateral. It extends in a round band—thus its name—down through the abdominal ring and attaches at the labia majora situated under the pubic symphysis. The uterus is also supported by the broad ligament which wraps over the uterus in a broad fold. It extends from the side of the uterus to the wall of the pelvis. (See Figure 2.)

This support or suspension by these two ligaments allows the uterus to grow and rise from a pelvic organ in its nonpregnant state to an abdominal organ. After 13-weeks gestation, as the uterus continues to grow and enlarge, it contacts the anterior abdominal wall and displaces the intestines laterally and superiorly (upwards). During the pregnancy, it continues to rise, ultimately, almost to the liver at 36-weeks gestation. (See Figure 3.)

The unique suspension by its ligaments that allows the uterus to rise is an important fact for you to know. When the woman is standing or sitting, the plane of the uterus corresponds to the plane of the pelvic outlet which allows the uterus to tilt forward. The muscles of the abdominal wall support the uterus in this plane. When the pregnant woman is supine, the uterus falls back and rests upon the vertebral column and the near-by great vessels, especially the inferior vena cava and the descending aorta. This creates a condition known as Supine Hypotensive Syndrome. (See the section on the Cardiovascular System and positioning on the table.)

By the end of 13 weeks when the uterus begins to enter the abdominal cavity, the pregnant woman will be able to feel the enlarging uterus with her hand over her abdomen. This will be an exciting discovery, for she will experience it as physical proof that she is really pregnant.

Figure 1

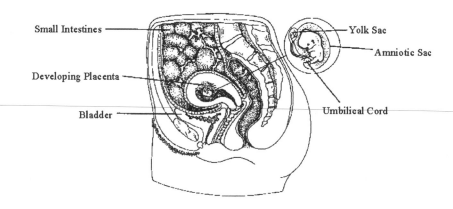

Small Intestines —

Developing Placenta —

Bladder —

Yolk Sac

Amniotic Sac

Umbilical Cord

Uterus at 6 weeks

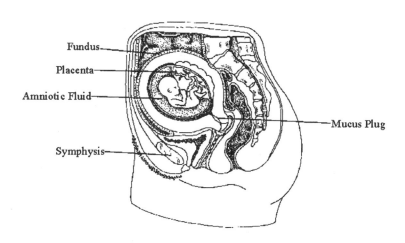

Fundus

Placenta

Amniotic Fluid

Symphysis

Mucus Plug

Uterus at 3 months

Reprinted with permission from The Growing Uterus Chart Series, Maternity Center Association, 48 East 92nd Street, New York, NY 10128.

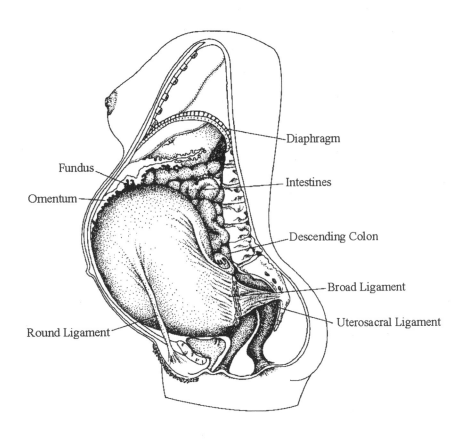

Figure 2

Round Ligament

Reprinted with permission from The Growing Uterus Chart Series, Maternity Center
Association, 48 East 92nd Street, New York, NY 10128.

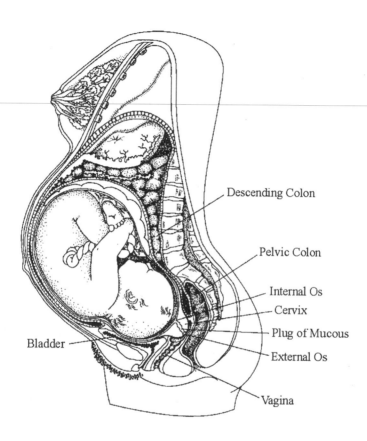

Figure 3

The uterus at 36 weeks gestation

Reprinted with permission from The Growing Uterus Chart Series, Maternity Center
Association, 48 East 92nd Street, New York, NY 10128.

CERVIX

The cervix is the opening into the uterus. Along with the uterus, the cervix also goes through some remarkable changes. A massage therapist need not be concerned about these changes. However, your client will be very aware of vaginal discharges. If she does any reading or attends childbirth education classes, she will be watching for changes in vaginal discharge.

As you can see by comparing the nonpregnant cervix shown in Figure 4 to the pregnant cervix shown in Figure 5, the glands of the cervix undergo marked growth by the end of the pregnancy. This growth takes up approximately ½ of the entire mass of the cervix. Its structure takes on a honeycomb appearance with winding and twisting surfaces. These meshes are filled with strong, gummy mucous.

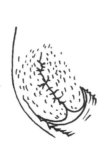
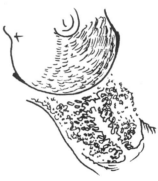

Figure 4
The nonpregnant cervix

Figure 5
The pregnant cervix

From Bobak, IM and Jensen, M.D.: Essentials of Maternity Nursing, 3rd edition, 1991, St. Louis, Mosby-Year Book, Inc.

These changes begin soon after pregnancy begins with the purpose of blocking and sealing the uterus. The baby (fetus) is enclosed within the membranes of the water bag and the cervical opening is sealed creating a sterile, safe place for the baby to grow and develop.

Sometime in the last few weeks of the woman's pregnancy, she will be looking for the "loss of her mucous plug." When it occurs, she will be excited, viewing this event as a visible sign that labor will begin soon. The only negative aspect of this event that you as a therapist will need to be aware of is the definition of "soon." "Soon" can mean several days to a couple of weeks. Your client will have a tendency to define "soon" as today or tonight. Your role, if she chooses to talk to you about the losing of her mucous plug, is to help with a realistic definition of "soon."

What does the loss of a mucous plug look like?

The mucous plug will look like clear, thick, gummy, sticky mucous. It may have streaks of pink or brown blood mixed in it. It may be expelled over a period of several days resulting in a stringy discharge. Or it may be expelled all at once and look like a large clump of sticky, gummy mucous. Large amounts of blood in any vaginal discharge needs to be evaluated by your client's physician or midwife.

Can she lose her mucous plug too early?

Any signs or symptoms of a mucous discharge before the beginning of the 8th month of pregnancy could be a symptom of early or preterm labor. If your client shares with you information about mucousy discharge before she is close to her expected date of confinement (EDC), instruct her to call her physician or midwife.

SKIN

Skin changes are one of the ways pregnancy is manifested by the woman's body. These changes will be very important to her. Do not overlook the connection of her body image and self-esteem that can impact on how she will view skin changes. Keep in mind that in this country, poor self-esteem in women is almost a chronic condition and poor self-esteem and poor body image usually go together. As her massage therapist you have the opportunity to help her deal with any negative feelings she might have associated with skin changes.

Stretch Marks

Called Striae Gravidarum, stretch marks usually appear in the later months of the pregnancy. They are reddish, slightly depressed streaks and are most common in the skin of the abdomen and sometimes in the skin of the breast and hips, buttocks and thighs.

These skin changes appear in approximately fifty percent of pregnant women. We do not know why some women do not have stretch marks. The color of the skin does not seem to make a difference, since women of all races and ethnic groups are prone to have stretch marks. Men, of course, who gain weight fast or lift weights that result in fast muscle growth may also develop stretch marks in the skin covering the muscle growth or the area of storage of extra weight.

We do not know what is present in the pregnant women who do not get stretch marks, it possibly is related to the amount of collagen in their skin. There are lotions and creams on the market advertised to help prevent stretch marks. In my experience, they do not work except perhaps to give the woman the satisfaction of something to do to try to prevent them. Lotions and creams that contain ingredients such as cocoa butter or aloe certainly promote optimal health of the skin and do no harm.

The good news that you will want to share with your client is that after the pregnancy the discolorations will fade usually to a silvery color. She will have to hunt for them in most cases in order to see them. (See Figure 6.)

If this is not the woman's first pregnancy, new stretch marks can be superimposed over old silvery marks. Your role is educating and reassuring her about how and why they appear and how they will fade after she has her baby. The fading process may take 3 or 4 months after delivery. I do not know of any technique or treatment to speed up the fading process.

It is appropriate also for the massage therapist to offer skin care information. The only skin product that the pregnant woman should not use is the anti-wrinkle cream that contains Retin-A. Retin-A creams were first introduced as a prescription treatment for badly scarred skin. Vitamin A taken in large amounts by mouth can cause birth defects in the baby. The amount of Vitamin A in cosmetic products containing Retin-A for applying to the skin will vary. There are no controls for absorption into the body through the skin. There is no way to predict or compensate for the client whose fear of getting stretch marks causes her to overuse a product. The over-the-counter product does not contain as much Retin-A as the prescription formula, but all the contraindications and adverse side effects apply.

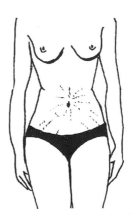

Figure 6

Stretch marks
Striae Gravidarum

Pigmentation Changes:
Linea Nigra and Melasma Gravidarum

Linea Nigra is pigmentation or darkening of the skin at the midline of the abdomen. A brownish-black line of color forms in all women, but especially in those women with brown or black hair. If the woman has not been pregnant before, she may be concerned when she notices its appearance.

She may also have irregular brownish patches of various sizes on her face and sometimes her neck, called "mask of pregnancy" or chloasma, also known as melasma gravidarum. Neither of these conditions are dangerous and will disappear after she has the baby. It is thought to be a result of the extra melanin (skin pigment) deposits created by increased estrogen and progesterone hormones produced by the pregnancy. We do not know what controls the site of their appearance—the midline of the abdomen and the face/neck area. Again the role of the therapist is one of reassurance that the condition is not dangerous and education about the resolution of the condition after she delivers her baby.

Cutaneous Vascular Changes

Spider Angioma, Spider Nevi, or angiomas, also called vascular spiders, will appear on the skin in about two thirds of Caucasian women and in about ten percent of Black women. These are minute, red marks on the skin with a center and tentacles branching out from the center. They most likely appear on the face, neck, upper chest, hands, and arms. They are caused by the extra estrogen produced by the pregnancy. Spider angiomas are harmless, but many times you will find your client asking about them with concern. (See Figure 7.)

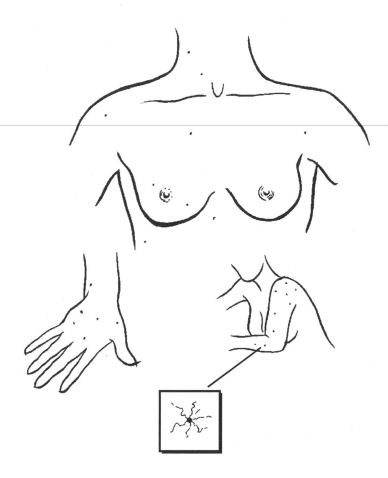

Figure 7

Spider Angioma
Spider Nevi

Palmar Erythema—blotchy red palms—also frequently appear in pregnant women, and with similar frequency as spider angioma. This condition is of no clinical significance and will disappear shortly after the woman delivers her baby.

Are there any skin changes your should be concerned about?

Yes. The pregnancy produces growth promoting agents that serve to increase the size of the uterus, cervix, breast, etc. On rare occasions these growth hormones can cause existing moles on the skin to begin to grow, or may cause new moles to appear. During pregnancy, the massage therapist can be most helpful in regularly inspecting any moles or freckles for changes. Any changes in color or size of a mole or the appearance of new moles should be shown to your client. Advise her to discuss these changes with her physician or midwife. Her medical provider may refer her to a dermatologist for evaluation.

Blood Flow To The Skin

Increased blood flow to the skin surface in pregnancy serves to dissipate excess heat generated by the increased metabolism of the pregnancy. Know that the pregnant woman is always going to be warmer than you are. You will need to take this into consideration when providing for a comfortable environment. You may find that if your pregnant client says the air conditioner is comfortable, it is sweater time for you. If she says she is hot or cold, listen to her and provide for as much temperature comfort as possible.

BREASTS

There are striking changes in the breasts as a result of pregnancy. Tenderness and tingling in the breasts are frequently the earliest sign of pregnancy. The pregnant woman will experience these changes within the first 2 months of her pregnancy. By the end of the 3rd month, enlargement and darkening of the nipples and the area (areola) around the nipples will occur. As in linea nigra and chloasma, the pigmentation will vary with the woman's complexion. It is more pink in blondes and darker in brunettes. (See Figure 8.)

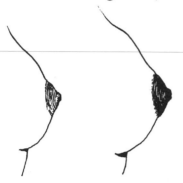

Figure 8

The nonpregnant and pregnant breast, nipple, and areola.

　　Scattered throughout the area of the areola are small elevations called Glands of Montgomery. These are sebaceous cysts that become enlarged. The breasts will continue to enlarge based on the woman's weight gain. Be aware that this may be a happy event, especially if she feels that her breasts are small. Notice, I am saying if she feels they are small. Her breast may not be small, but if she perceives them to be, they might as well be small. Again this has to do with her own body image. For the woman more endowed, breast enlargement can be perceived as a negative event. Excessive enlargement can result in stretch marks (striae). The skin of the breasts will take on a translucence, resulting in delicate tracing of visible veins.

　　Colostrum can appear as early as 2 months. Colostrum is the first food material produced by the breasts of a pregnant woman and is a function of her body preparing to nurture and feed her baby. It is high in protein and acts as a laxative for the newborn. It also contains a high concentration of antibodies to fight against many bacterial infections.

Should the massage therapist massage the breasts during pregnancy?

No. Stimulation of the breast and nipples in the pregnant woman is absolutely contraindicated. It is well documented in scientific literature that stimulation of the breasts and nipples causes the release of the hormone oxytocin. This hormone creates contractions of the uterus. Nipple stimulation has been demonstrated to cause extended or tetantic contractions lasting several minutes. These kinds of contractions do not routinely cause the cervix to begin to open or dilate, but long extended periods of the uterus squeezing on the baby can decrease circulation of the blood to the baby—thus decreasing oxygen and food nutrients—creating stress to the baby, especially if a portion of the cord is pressing on a bony baby part such as a shoulder or head.

I do not feel it is necessary for the massage therapist to understand the physiology of lactation. However, it is important for the therapist to understand that in many women certain stimulations can cause her to leak colostrum during the pregnancy, e.g., sexual arousal or hearing a baby cry. This can be embarrassing for her. If this happens to her, she may be too embarrassed to discuss it with her medical caretakers. If she chooses to confide in the therapist, the therapist should assure her that this event is normal in a lot of women, thus, helping her to accept that part of her body's normal reaction to pregnancy.

The same rule applies to the postpartum period (period of time that begins with the delivery of the baby and placenta and ends 6 weeks later). Stimulation of the breasts will release the hormone oxytocin. Since the postpartum woman is no longer pregnant, there is no danger to her fetus. However, any undue stimulation of the breasts will trigger the milk let-down response and can be embarrassing or uncomfortable to the breast feeding woman. And in the woman who is attempting to interrupt lactation, massage stimulation can promote the continuation of lactation or milk production.

ABDOMINAL WALL

The abdominal wall muscles, the abdominis recti, exposed to the extra tension of the growing uterus separate in the midline creating a condition called diastasis, meaning separation. This condition results in a severe loss of muscle tone. Some books say this happens occasionally, but in my experience it happens to most women to some degree. It can be severe in some women, especially in the mother who has had several pregnancies and may not have been educated about corrective exercises to regain muscle tone. During pregnancy, it can be so severe that a large portion of the anterior uterine wall is covered by only a layer of skin, fascia, and peritoneum. (See Figure 9.)

Closure of the separation during the 6 weeks after delivery (postpartum period) is important. Failure to regain good muscle tone can result in malpresentations such as feet-first or buttocks-first (breech) presentations or the baby lying crossways (transverse lie). The woman with either of these conditions will be facing delivery of her baby by a surgical procedure called cesarean birth. Cesarean deliveries are considered major surgery, and carry with them all the inherent risks associated with major surgery.

After delivery the abdominal walls will be flabby, and all women will have some diastasis recti. Checking for this condition during the postpartum period, and teaching the postpartum woman how to regain her muscle tone is an important part of your therapeutic hands-on care. (See Figure 10.)

Also, be aware that the postpartum woman's medical provider may not check for this condition or take the time to teach her corrective exercises. How to check your client for diastasis recti after her delivery, and the corrective exercise, is detailed in Chapter Six.

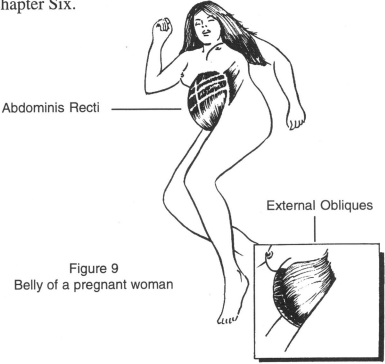

Abdominis Recti

External Obliques

Figure 9
Belly of a pregnant woman

Figure 10
Diastasis (Separation) of the abdominis recti.

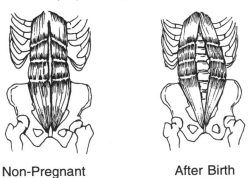

Non-Pregnant   After Birth

PROGRESSIVE LORDOSIS

Progressive lordosis is a characteristic feature of normal pregnancy. As a result of compensation for the anterior position of the enlarging uterus, the lordosis shifts the center of gravity back over the lower extremities.

There is increased mobility of the sacroiliac, sacrococcygeal, and the pubic joints during the pregnancy thought to be a result of hormonal changes of estrogen and progesterone. This shift alters the woman's posture, in turn causing discomfort in the lower portion of the back. This condition worsens later in the pregnancy. (See Figure 11.)

Figure 11

Lordosis as a result of the shift of the center of gravity.

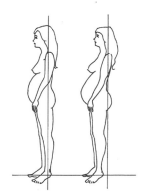

During the last trimester of pregnancy, aching, numbness, and weakness in the upper extremities are occasionally experienced. This is probably a result of the marked lordosis with anterior flexion of the neck and slumping of the shoulder girdle, which in turn produces traction on the ulnar and median nerves in the upper extremities. *(Williams Obstetrics.)*

As a result of the shift described above your client may have: low back pain; pain and instability in the hips; or aching, numbness, and weakness in the arms. Massage will help to alleviate these common discomforts. Awareness of the weakness and numbness in the arms allows you to be a source of reassurance.

In addition to massaging away sore muscles and tension, you can also teach the pregnant woman how to do the pelvic tilt to help alleviate low back pain. The pelvic tilt can be done standing, sitting, lying down, and on hands and knees. (See Figure 12.)

One caution when teaching pregnant women to do the pelvic tilt. The hands and knees position, with the excessive weight of the pregnant uterus pulling downward from the force of gravity, may cause back strain. Cautioning your clients to keep their backs straight while on hands and knees will avoid low back strain.

It is not a good idea to teach your client to do the pelvic tilt while lying supine. In this position the uterus falls back and rests on the vertebral column and the nearby great vessels, especially the vena cava and descending aorta.

Figure 12

The Pelvic Tilt
Standing
Hands and Knees

METABOLIC CHANGES

Metabolic changes refer to those changes that govern how the body processes digested food or nutrients—energy use at the cell level. In response to the fast-growing fetus, uterus, and placenta, and their increasing demands, the pregnant woman undergoes intense and numerous changes in energy demands. These changes manifest themselves in the form of weight gain.

Most of the weight gain in pregnancy is attributed to the increase in uterine size, the contents of the uterus, the breasts, and the increase in blood volume, extravascular and extracellular fluid.

The range of weight gain varies. Midwives place great emphasis on good nutrition which shows up as good weight gain. As a midwife, I want my pregnant clients to have gained at least 10 pounds by the end of the 20th week or 5-months gestation, and then to gain a pound a week. This amounts to approximately 30 to 35 pounds weight gain. If the woman starts out her pregnancy overweight, less weight gain is acceptable.

Nutritional needs

There are hundreds of books on the subject of nutrition in pregnancy. It is not within the scope of this work to prepare the massage therapist to act as a nutritional counselor to pregnant women. Her nutritional needs in terms of increased food, vitamins, and minerals is best left in the hands of her prenatal caregiver—physician/midwife. (See Figure 13.)

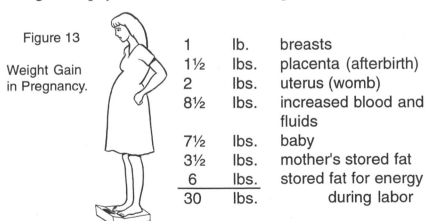

Figure 13

Weight Gain
in Pregnancy.

1	lb.	breasts
1½	lbs.	placenta (afterbirth)
2	lbs.	uterus (womb)
8½	lbs.	increased blood and fluids
7½	lbs.	baby
3½	lbs.	mother's stored fat
6	lbs.	stored fat for energy
30	lbs.	during labor

However, the massage therapist needs to know that the pregnant woman will have an increased appetite and will be gaining weight. If she has a poor body image concept, she may find gaining weight disturbing. She may see herself as getting fat rather than gaining the weight needed to grow a healthy baby.

Over and over in my practice, I find women who worry about "getting fat and ugly" when pregnant. They tell me things like, "my husband (boyfriend) tells me I am fat." Some of this is related to poor self-esteem in women, and some of it is related to the fact that we never see anywhere—television, movies, magazines—pictures of women who are pregnant and look sexy.

Do you remember the controversy about Demi Moore posing while very pregnant for *Vanity Fair* magazine? In the small town where I live, the issue was pulled from the shelf. I had to travel to a large mall in a nearby town to find a copy. The next year there was hardly a media blink when she appeared on the same magazine cover nude and nonpregnant. Even the advertisers in the *Lamaze Parents' Magazine* over the years have dropped the use of photographs of pregnant women in lace gowns and robes, showing bare pregnant bellies and breasts. They now choose to use more abstract photos and the mother/baby Madonna images.

This is not a forum for teaching both men and women that women have body hair, women's breast are not necessarily pointed, and that the pregnant woman is not fat. However, the massage therapist can play an important role in helping the pregnant client deal with any negative body image problems she shares. Also, be aware that if she discusses body image issues with the massage therapist, she may be looking for an empathetic listener rather than advice or any solution to the problem.

Water Metabolism

Edema or water retention is a normal physiological alteration of pregnancy. Water retention is a result of a resetting of osmotic thresholds for thirst and hormone secretions affecting the kidneys. At term the water content of the fetus, placenta, and amniotic fluid is about 3.5 liters. Approximately 3.0 liters of water accumulates in the maternal blood volume and in the increased size of the uterus and breasts, making the average water retention in the full-term pregnant woman about 6.5 liters.

Studies have shown that the woman who has some swelling of her hands and feet during pregnancy will have a healthier baby than the woman who has none. Excessive retention of water, with the development of severe edema of lower limbs, hands, and face, is usually present in pregnancy induced hypertension or toxemia.

A good rule of thumb about edema: normal edema of pregnancy is that which accumulates in the woman's feet, legs, and hands as the day progresses and reaches its greatest amount at the end of the day before she goes to bed. After a normal night of rest, most of the edema is gone. This edema is the result of increased venous pressure below the level of the uterus as a result of partial obstruction or occlusion of the vena cava by the enlarging pregnant uterus and the pull of gravity.

Abnormal edema is that which is found by the pregnant woman upon arising in the morning after a night of rest. Instead of less swelling than when she went to bed, she has more. Usually this dangerous type of edema is manifested by swelling in the rest of her body, especially the face, as well as in the lower extremities. Along with the abnormal edema of toxemia, a pregnant woman can have high blood pressure. High blood pressure is a contraindication for massage.

It is not the role of the massage therapist to distinguish between normal (pathologic) or abnormal (nonpathologic) swelling. Even if the therapist has the skills to measure blood pressure with a blood pressure cuff (sphygmomanometer), it is not recommended. As we note in the section on cardiovascular changes, normal blood pressure in the pregnant woman varies greatly.

A safe way to handle clients with edema is to ask them if their swelling has been noted by their physician or midwife. If so, ask them what their physician/midwife advised about the swelling. Also, if you are not sure, you can always call the medical caretaker and discuss your concerns.

Fat Metabolism

Fat metabolism in pregnancy is increased. A pregnant woman will have increased cholesterol and other fats (lipids) in the blood. She will store fat more readily especially during the second trimester. It is felt the extra fat stores make available extra energy for use during the labor—labor being a time in which she may go many hours without the desire or ability to eat.

HEMATOMOLOGIC (BLOOD) CHANGES

Blood volume increases in all pregnant women and in some women this increase can be nearly double. The reason for this increased blood volume is the enlarging uterus. This increase meets the demands of the enlarged uterus and its greatly increased veins and arteries which need to nourish themselves. The increased blood volume also serves to protect the mother and fetus against the harmful effects of decreased blood return to the heart while she is in the erect and supine positions. It also protects the mother against the ill effects of blood loss associated with too much bleeding at the time of birth.

The pregnant woman's blood volume begins to increase in the first trimester, rises much faster in the second trimester and tapers off in the last trimester. The increase is made up of plasma and red blood cells.

THE CARDIOVASCULAR SYSTEM

The pulse rate increases by about 10 to 15 beats per minute. Cardiac output, or amount of blood pumped by the heart at rest, increases in the first trimester and remains elevated during the rest of the pregnancy. Cardiac output is higher when the woman is in the lateral recumbent position (lying on her side) than when she is supine.

As the diaphragm is elevated by the enlarging uterus, the heart is displaced to the left and upward. At the same time, it is rotated to the side on its long axis. As a result of this rotation, and the slight enlargement of the heart associated with its increased work handling the increased blood volume, the x-rays of a pregnant woman can mimic some heart disease processes.

Because of the increase in the blood volume, up to ninety percent of women will have a change in heart sounds, referred to as a heart murmur. These changes would be considered abnormal in the nonpregnant woman, but are usually considered benign in the normal healthy pregnant woman.

It is not the role of the massage therapist to diagnose or evaluate the heart. However, any cardiac abnormalities need to be a part of your history. It would not be uncommon for your pregnant client to tell you that her physician or midwife told her she had a heart murmur. If this happens, clarify with your client or her medical caretaker if indeed this is a normal physiologic event associated with the pregnancy rather than a pre-existing heart disease process.

Another important aspect of the prenatal client is that generally she is young and can be expected to be in good health. In the population past childbearing age, this cannot be assumed.

What happens in the supine position?

A pregnant woman placed in the supine position may become dizzy or even pass out on your table. In the supine position, the large pregnant uterus compresses the venous system that returns blood from the lower half of the body. Cardiac filling from blood returned via the vena cava slows and causes decreased cardiac output. If the blood is not returned to the heart, there is none present to be pumped no matter how good the pump (heart) works. (See Figure 14.)

This condition is referred to as Supine Hypotensive Syndrome. The pregnant woman may experience this event as dizziness while lying on her back. Whether she experiences dizziness or not the event still occurs. *Williams Obstetrics* says that this event increases blood pressure in the femoral venous system especially below the area of the compression, but it does not change blood pressure when taken in the arm.

Therefore, taking the woman's blood pressure is not a reliable evaluation of the pressure in the arteries that lie distal or below the compressed area.

Placing a pregnant women in the supine position to perform massage any time after the end of the first trimester is always contraindicated. The following list outlines exactly what happens to her and how it involves other organs and systems.

1. The uterus compresses the inferior vena cava, decreasing blood return to the heart.

2. Decreased blood return to the heart makes less blood available for the heart to pump.

3. Reduction in cardiac output decreases blood flow to the kidneys.

4. Reduction in blood flow to the kidneys results in decreased sodium and water excretion.

5. Decrease in sodium and water excretion results in increased edema.

6. Increased edema results in development of varicose veins in legs, vulva, and vaginal wall.

7. The uterus compresses the aorta decreasing the amount of oxygenated blood available to the uterine artery.

8. Compressed aorta creates up to a three-fold increase in femoral blood pressure (not measurable with a blood pressure cuff).

9. Increase in femoral blood pressure contributes to the development of varicose veins in legs, vulva, and vaginal wall.

10. Decreased blood to the uterine artery causes decrease in amount of oxygen and food nutrient to the fetus.

11. Decreased oxygen and food to the fetus causes stress in the fetus.

12. In the supine position, the uterus compresses the uterers of the kidneys at the pelvic brim contributing to enlarged and convoluted (twisted and folded) ureters which in extreme cases can damage the kidneys.

13. Less blood pumped affects every part of the woman's body including her brain, causing dizziness.

14. Dizziness experienced by the pregnant woman will be frightening and may result in her losing consciousness.

Many of these events described above occur whether or not the woman experiences dizziness. Dizziness is a sign that the above described events are severe. If this happens to your client, have her sit up which will correct the problem. Reassure her with an explanation of what is happening.

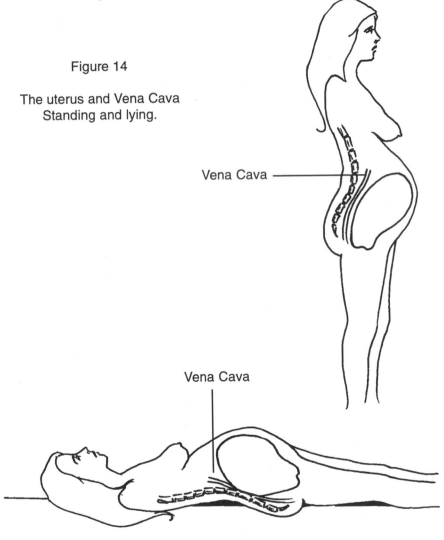

Figure 14

The uterus and Vena Cava
Standing and lying.

Vena Cava

Vena Cava

From Bobak, IM and Jensen, M.D.: Essentials of Maternity Nursing, 3rd edition, 1991, St. Louis, Mosby-Year Book, Inc.

In Chapter Nine on prenatal massage routine, correct body alignment to prevent Supine Hypotensive Syndrome on the massage table and massage techniques are explained in detail. The above described physiologic changes in the pregnant woman as a result of lying in the supine position provide the rationale for and the importance of the technique changes.

When do you stop placing your pregnant clients in the supine position for massage?

Figure 15 shows serial changes in antecubital and femoral venous blood pressure throughout normal pregnancy and early postpartum of women in the supine position. As you can see the difference in the normal pressure for a pregnant woman is quite dramatic when she is put in the supine position. By the middle of the 2nd trimester, the pressure increase has doubled and has tripled by the end of the 3rd trimester.

At the beginning of 13-weeks gestation, the uterus becomes an abdominal organ. At that time the supine position allows the uterus to fall back upon the pelvic brim causing a significant blood pressure rise in the femoral vein. Play it safe, if you know a woman is pregnant, do not place her in the supine position at any stage of pregnancy.

Figure 15
Graph showing femoral blood pressure rise in supine position.

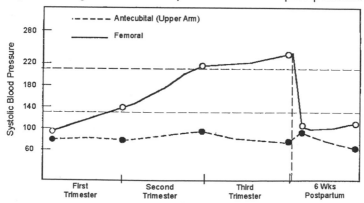

Should I advise my pregnant clients not to lie or sleep in the supine position?

No. It is my experience that most women assume a side-lying position for sleeping, especially as the pregnancy progresses. Her comfort level for reclining and lying will determine her sleep position. I feel the body has an innate or natural wisdom of its own that will not allow a pregnant woman to assume a sleep position that is harmful to her. The massage therapist advising a client not to sleep on her back can create unnecessary anxiety, especially if she awakens to find herself in the supine position.

DEEP VENOUS THROMBOSIS

An absolute contraindication for massage of the pregnant woman.

As discussed in Chapter Six, pregnancy increases the risk of deep vein thrombosis (DVT) or blood clots in the lower extremities. *Williams Obstetrics* says, "the likelihood of deep venous thrombosis in the normal pregnancy and the postpartum period is increased by a factor of five when compared to non-pregnant women of similar age." Deep venous thrombosis and the life-threatening pulmonary embolism that can result from this condition, is a major cause of death during pregnancy in this country. Pulmonary embolism is a condition caused by small blood clots in other parts of the body breaking and floating loose in the blood stream and lodging in the lungs creating a life-threatening medical emergency

Up until the 1950s deep vein thrombosis of the lower extremity was seen mostly in women in the postpartum period. Early ambulation and avoiding bed rest even in women delivered by cesarean has resulted in a dramatic decrease of the problem in the postpartum period. So much so that now the incidence of deep vein thrombosis is greater in the prenatal period. This is not a common problem and I do not want to unduly alarm therapists. *Williams Obstetrics* states there is probably an incidence of one to two in 1000 pregnancies. However, massage in the presence of deep vein clots in the lower extremities can result in small clots breaking loose, traveling in the blood stream, and lodging in the lungs—pulmonary embolism.

Women at greater risk to develop DVT during pregnancy are women who have used oral contraceptives (birth control pills) before becoming pregnant and women who work at a job that requires sitting for long periods of time. The symptoms of DVT are an abrupt onset of severe pain and edema, and heat and redness of the leg and thigh. Usually this condition involves most of the deep venous system from the foot to the iliofemoral region. However, some women can have a dangerous amount of deep vein clots with little reaction in the way of pain, abnormal heat, or swelling. This is all the more reason for the massage therapists to make the following techniques a part of their massage management of the pregnant client.

Professional management of the risk of deep vein thrombosis in the pregnant client.

The history form used at the first visit should include the following questions:

- Have you taken birth control pills in the past year before becoming pregnant?
- Do you work at a job that requires sitting for long periods of time?

If the answer to either of these questions is YES, you should note that the woman is at risk for developing DVT.

If your client is at risk for DVT, a simple assessment at the beginning of the massage and documentation of negative findings at this assessment is absolutely indicated. A prudent massage therapist will add this assessment to the massage technique with every pregnant client.

At the beginning of the massage, the woman is placed in the supine position with a pillow or rolled towel placed under her right side tilting her 15 to 20 degrees to the left side to avoid Supine Hypotensive Syndrome. With her legs straight, using both hands on each side of her leg, palpate each extremity for tenderness and abnormal heat. Next stretch the Achilles tendon on both extremities (Homan's sign) by placing the leg straight on your table. Apply gentle pressure on the knee, keeping the leg straight. With the other hand, firmly flex the foot toward the woman's chin. The sign is positive if this maneuver creates any pain in the leg. (See Figure 16.)

A positive Homan's sign could be due to benign conditions such as a bruise or muscle strain. However, in the presence of tenderness, abnormal heat, or a positive Homan's sign, massage should be postponed and the client referred to her medical provider for evaluation.

Figure 16

How to check
Homan's Sign

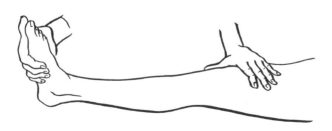

RESPIRATORY TRACT

Anatomical changes associated with the rising level of the diaphragm (up to 4 cm) during pregnancy create an increase in the thoracic circumference of about 6 cm. The subcostal angle widens appreciably as the transverse diameter of the thoracic cage increases (2 cm). These changes allow for the increased oxygen needs of the mother and fetus. (See Figure 17.)

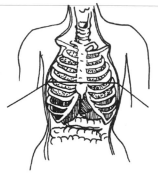

Figure 17

Anatomical rise of the diaphragm during pregnancy.

Resetting of oxygen needs in the body by the hormone progesterone changes the respiratory rate very little. However, even in early pregnancy, an increased awareness of the desire to breathe in the pregnant woman is common. She may find that she is sighing frequently. She may feel that she is experiencing shortness of breath. This feeling of shortness of breath can be frightening to her. Encourage her to discuss her symptoms with her physician or midwife.

GASTROINTESTINAL TRACT

As the pregnancy progresses the stomach and intestines are displaced laterally by the growing uterus. The hormones produced by the pregnancy have a slowing effect on smooth muscle and the pregnant woman will have decreased tone and motility of the entire gastrointestinal tract. This means it takes longer for the stomach to empty and for the intestinal contents to travel to evacuation. (See Figure 3.)

Heartburn (Pyrosis), common in most pregnancies, is caused by a reflux of acidic secretions into the lower esophagus. The altered position of the stomach probably contributes to its frequency.

Why is displacement of intestinal organs, especially the appendix, important to know?

Intestinal organ displacement changes physical findings. In pregnancy the appendix can be hard to pinpoint anatomically even for the physician. Heat applied to appendicitis can result in a ruptured appendix and life-threatening peritonitis. Because of this displacement, heat or hot packs applied to the abdomen or flank is contraindicated in the pregnant woman.

Mouth

Excessive salivation called ptylism occurs in some women, especially Black women and women with origins in the Mediterranean area. This can be a very uncomfortable and distressing event, with the woman spitting quarts of fluid in a day. Ptylism is usually experienced in the first few months of pregnancy and can accompany nausea and vomiting. Ptylism can also exacerbate or worsen the severity of nausea and vomiting.

The gums of the pregnant woman may become softened and have an increase in blood in their tissue. This can result in bleeding gums even when mildly traumatized. Some women will have a large amount of swelling of the gums—epulis of pregnancy. These gum changes return to normal spontaneously shortly after delivery.

It was once thought that tooth loss in the pregnant woman was inevitable. There is no good evidence that pregnancy causes tooth decay if good dental hygiene is followed.

Gallbladder

Gallbladder function is slowed in pregnancy. The gallbladder can become distended and hypotonic and the bile production thicken. It is commonly accepted by physicians and midwives that pregnancy predisposes a woman to the formation of gallstones.

I do not feel that this will have much bearing on your work as massage therapists, but you should know that any pain in the upper right quadrant of the abdomen can be from inflammation of the gallbladder. The pain can range from mild to unbearable. Any work you might do to alleviate a woman's symptoms certainly would do no harm. Teaching her how to stimulate the gallbladder by massaging the acupressure point between the thumb and the forefinger—Large Intestine 4 (LI4) also referred to as Hoku—many times will give her relief. (See Figure 22 for location of L14.)

Liver

There is no evidence of any distinct changes that take place in the liver associated with pregnancy. *(Williams Obstetrics.)*

Hemorrhoids

The occurrence of hemorrhoids whether pregnant or not is associated with constipation. The problem is worse in pregnancy due to generalized slowing of smooth muscle—intestines are smooth muscle. Also, compression of the large bowel by the growing uterus makes constipation a real threat. This coupled with the edema and congestion caused by the elevated pressure in the veins below the level of the uterus is a major contributing cause of hemorrhoids.

Any advice to your pregnant client about constipation should be limited to identification of foods high in fiber, use of psysillum seed, and encouraging increased fluids. Refer her to her physician/midwife for advice about laxatives and stool softeners.

ENDOCRINE SYSTEM

Some of the most important changes of pregnancy have to do with hormones produced by the endocrine system—ceasing of ovulation, growth of the fetus, and milk production. The production changes of the endocrine system do not impact your practice. I have chosen to deal with these changes in other areas of this chapter, e.g., the section on breasts.

RENAL SYSTEM (URINARY TRACT)

Kidney

Bear in mind that the changes we are discussing are normal changes as a result of pregnancy—pregnancy defined as a normal physiologic condition, not a disease. The disease process of the renal system can be greatly increased as a result of pregnancy.

Remarkable changes in the structure and function of the kidneys and ureters occur as a result of pregnancy. The kidney itself increases only slightly in size. However, the flow of blood to the kidney and the filtration rate of the kidney is increased. These changes begin early in the pregnancy rising to a fifty percent increase by the beginning of the second trimester (14 weeks).

Renal function studies on pregnant women show that urinary functions are affected to a large degree by the supine position. In the supine position blood flow to the kidney is decreased considerably. *(Williams Obstetrics.)* As discussed earlier this is a result of reduced venous return to the heart which results from obstruction of the vena cava and the iliac veins by the enlarging pregnant uterus when in supine position.

Ureters

After the growing uterus rises completely out of the pelvis, it rests upon the ureters, compressing them at the pelvic brim. As a result of this phenomenon, most women will have typical ureteral dilatation above the pelvic brim, but more so on the right side. It is felt that this is a result of the cushioning effect provided on the left by the sigmoid colon and also by a greater compression of the right ureter as a consequence of the normal dextrorotation of the enlarging uterus.

As noted earlier the hormones of pregnancy tend to slow the action of smooth muscles. The ureters are made of smooth muscle and the normal peristalsis, or downward wave-like motion, is slowed. As a result of this the ureters can become elongated or lengthen and become enfolded upon themselves or convoluted. These are normal changes, creating no problems and the ureters return to their normal size and length by six-to eight-weeks postpartum unless infection happens.

Bladder

The bladder enlarges during pregnancy causing it to thicken, thus decreasing its volume. The pressure inside the bladder increases as does the pressure of the urethra. These pressure changes are to compensate for the increased pressure of the enlarging uterus and preserve urinary continence—in other words so that the woman will be able to hold her urine.

The most common problem in the pregnant woman is a bladder infection. In my experience almost all the pregnant women who experience recurring bladder infections do not drink enough water. This problem can also occur because of poor nutrition and personal hygiene habits—wiping from back to front after urination or a bowel movement.

The most common problem that will impact on your work with the pregnant woman is urinary frequency. During the first 3 months of pregnancy the uterus is anteflexed and leaning against the bladder. As the growing uterus rises out of the pelvis in the beginning of the 14th week, the pressure on the bladder is relieved, only to return in the latter weeks of the pregnancy. (See Figures 1 and 3.)

In the woman having her first baby, the baby's head will drop into the pelvis (engage) sometime several weeks before labor starts. This causes pressure on the bladder from the weight of the contents of the uterus.

Why does this impact on your massage technique?

A pregnant woman may need to empty her bladder frequently. If you are doing a full-body massage taking an hour or so, you need to offer her the opportunity to go to the bathroom sometime during the session, perhaps at the time of a position change on the table. She may not experience the need to urinate, but you need to be sensitive to this possibility and offer the bathroom break.

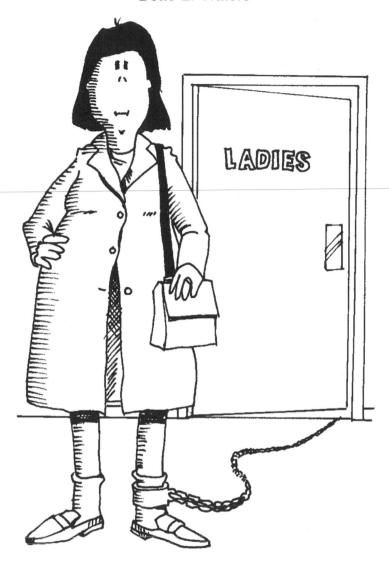

I used to worry about my credit limit...now I
worry about my bladder limit.

Chapter Two

DISCOMFORTS OF PREGNANCY

The list of discomforts of pregnancy can be long, and symptoms can vary from person to person. This chapter addresses the common discomforts experienced by most pregnant women. They have been selected because the techniques of the massage therapist offer solutions more than likely not available to the pregnant female in traditional maternity care.

NAUSEA

The nausea and vomiting associated with early pregnancy is so prevalent that it is considered one of the first signs of pregnancy. We do not understand what causes nausea in pregnancy. The medical textbooks offer little information about how to treat or control this problem. *Williams Obstetrics*, a 900-page book, offers a half page on nausea of pregnancy and most of the half page talks about the different theories of why women experience nausea. In a separate chapter, three paragraphs discuss nausea with severe vomiting, called hyperemesis gravidarium, which many times requires hospital intervention with intravenous fluids.

I am not being critical of the medical literature. The point I wish to make is that medicine does not consider the debilitating effects of common nausea and vomiting of pregnancy as anything serious. Many times women simply view nausea and vomiting of pregnancy as a normal condition and just "live with it."

This attitude was vividly demonstrated to me recently. My bright and beautiful 19-year-old granddaughter, pregnant, experiencing many hours of daily nausea and vomiting, losing weight, pale with dark circles under her eyes, said to me, when I chided her for not calling me, her midwife grandmother, for help, "I just thought it was normal."

It is normal, meaning it is not the result of a disease process. However, there are ways to resolve or decrease the discomforts associated with the nausea and vomiting of pregnancy. The methods I share with you are safe for a massage therapist to recommend to a pregnant client. The first method I call "Eating Regimen for Nausea of Pregnancy." I cannot take credit for this regimen. It was taught to me in my midwifery education program, and comes from Varney's *Midwifery* textbook. However, I can attest to its effectiveness having used it with good results for more than eleven years in my practice as a nurse-midwife.

The regimen begins at bedtime:

1. Drink a glass of juice with 2 teaspoons of sugar (this is the only time I ever deliberately instruct a pregnant woman to eat sugar). There is something about the sugar that helps keep a woman's blood sugar levels up during the night.

2. Place dry crackers by the bedside and upon awakening in the morning, eat several dry crackers before getting out of bed.

3. Get up slowly. Go immediately to the kitchen and eat something. It does not matter what. Worry about good nutrition later in the pregnancy after the nausea and vomiting have resolved.

4. Eat something every 2 hours throughout the day and finish the eating regimen with the glass of juice and sugar at bedtime.

Acupressure wristbands are another very effective method for control of nausea. Many midwives recommend acupressure wristbands with excellent results. Few physicians seem to know about this method. However, this method was first studied by an obstetrician, Dr. J. W. Dundee, "P6 Acupressure Reduces Morning Sickness," and published in the *Journal of the Royal Society of Medicine*, August 1988, (a British journal). Elisabeth Hyde, a nurse-midwife at Yale University repeated the study and published the results of her work, "Acupressure Therapy For Morning Sickness," in the *Journal of Nurse-Midwifery* in 1989.

Acupressure bands are elastic wristbands with a plastic button attached. The plastic button is placed on the wrist and applies constant pressure on the energy meridian identified as Pericardium Six or P6. (See Figure 18.) The bands are packaged with pictures demonstrating how to wear them and where the P6 acupressure point is located. They are marketed under different names. Seabands or QueasyAide are names that are sold at most chain drugstores and discount stores such as Walgrens and Walmart. The instructions for use usually refer to carsickness, airsickness, or seasickness, rather than for the control of the nausea of pregnancy. It has been my experience that the acupressure bands work well and many times offer relief when all else fails. It is a safe method for the massage therapist to recommend.

Figure 18
Pericardium 6 (P6)

Acupressure point for control
of nausea.

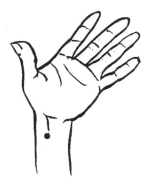

A commonly overlooked companion of severe nausea and vomiting is a condition called ptyalism (pronounced ti'-ah-lizm). Ptyalism is a condition of excessive secretion of saliva. This condition is seen in the early weeks of pregnancy for Black women or women with Mediterranean ethnic roots. This condition is recognized by saliva in amounts that are impossible to swallow, and many times requires the carrying of a container for expectoration (spitting). It has been my experience that control of the excessive salivation dramatically reduces the nausea and vomiting symptoms.

There is an old wives' folk remedy for control of ptyalism that I learned from the pregnant Haitian women I cared for in my practice in Florida. There is no scientific data available about this remedy or why it works, but it works.

Advise the pregnant woman to purchase fresh parsley. After washing it thoroughly, break it into two- or three-inch sprigs and place it in a small plastic bag convenient for carrying around with her. Every five minutes she is to chew a sprig of parsley and then expectorate (spit out) the chewed residuals rather than swallow them. Recommending this regimen to your pregnant client with severe nausea associated with excessive salivation is safe, and can certainly do no harm. If it solves her problem, she will think you are a genius.

Severe nausea and vomiting, unresponsive to the above interventions, many times has a psychological component that includes some underlying conflict within a woman's relationships—usually unrecognized by the pregnant woman. This is identified as hyperemesis gravidarium and is a problem that requires medical intervention to establish normal electrolyte balance and adequate hydration. This treatment is usually carried out in a hospital. Conflict resolution is an area the massage therapist is not educated to handle, and should not be attempted as part of a therapeutic massage program.

Finally, nausea and vomiting of pregnancy is self-limiting and usually begins to subside at the end of the first trimester. Your pregnant client may or may not gain weight during this time. However, the fetus is quite small and does not require large amounts of energy. Unchecked weight loss as a result of nausea and vomiting of pregnancy is a problem for the medical provider.

FATIGUE

The first trimester is also a time when the pregnant woman experiences fatigue. She generally feels tired and needs longer periods of sleep. As with nausea this is a self-limiting condition and usually disappears at the end of her 3rd or 4th month. My advice for this problem is to encourage her to listen to the wisdom of her body. If her body says to sleep, then sleep.

ROUND LIGAMENT PAIN

We discussed in Chapter One how the round ligament suspends and supports the uterus allowing it to rise from a pelvic organ to an abdominal organ in the section on physiology.

As you can see in Figure 2 the round ligaments attach on both sides of the uterus just below and in front of the fallopian tubes, pass through the abdominal musculature at the inguinal canal, and insert in the upper portion of the labia majora just below the symphysis pubis. This ligament along with the uterosacral ligament is what suspends the uterus, allowing it to rise from a pelvic organ to an abdominal organ. The tissue of the round ligament is made up of the same tissue as the uterus and has the ability to contract.

Sudden movements on the part of the woman can trigger a painful spasm or contraction of this ligament. The spasm is usually experienced as a sudden onset of sharp pain in the lower abdomen on one side or the other, and many times will radiate down into the groin area. It can last five minutes or more. If the pregnant woman does not know about round ligament pain, this can be a frightening experience. Most likely her reaction will be to assume that anything that hurts as much as round ligament spasm, means something is wrong.

It is not the role of the massage therapist to distinguish between any pain the pregnant woman may have in the abdomen. However, it is appropriate for the therapist to teach her about round ligament pain and encourage her to ask her physician or midwife about her symptoms.

If a pregnant client tells you her physician/midwife says her discomfort is round ligament pain, some comfort measures include:

1. Flex her knees toward her abdomen until the pain subsides.

2. Soak in a warm bath.

3. Support the abdomen with a pillow and put a pillow between her legs when lying on her side.

4. Attempt to avoid sudden movements (rise slowly from sitting position; sit slowly).

5. Turn to side-lying and push herself up with arms and elbows from a lying position. (See Figure 19.)

Figure 19

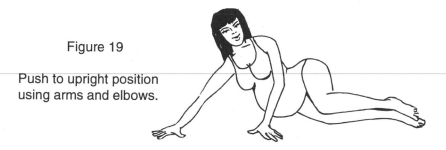

Push to upright position
using arms and elbows.

Do not advise her to apply heat. Heat applied to this type of pain is contraindicated without knowing for sure there is no medical complication such as appendicitis. Heat applied to the abdomen in the case of appendicitis could make the condition worse. The therapist is not educated to make this type of differentiation.

HEARTBURN

Heartburn is a burning sensation in the midline of the chest between the breasts or higher. It is called heartburn because the sensation is experienced as being close to the heart. It is caused by the acid contents of the stomach backing up into the esophagus. The stomach and digestive tract are hollow organs and their walls are made of smooth muscle. The hormones produced by the pregnancy have a slowing effect on the normal wave-like progression of the alternate contraction and relaxation of the muscle fibers that act to propel stomach contents along the digestive tract (peristalsis).

Women may experience heartburn as early as the first trimester. By the time the pregnant woman reaches the third trimester, the slowing of peristalsis is further complicated by the enlarging uterus displacing the stomach and the intestines. (See Figure 3.) She may find that the problem is worse when in bed.

Heartburn can be decreased by eating smaller, more frequent meals. She may take Tums. Tums is calcium carbonate which acts as an antacid and also is an excellent source of calcium. Liquid antacids and Rolaids contain aluminum hydroxide and magnesium, which can interfere with her body's ability to absorb iron and vitamins, and should be taken only upon the advice of her medical provider. At night placing an extra pillow under her head and torso may also help with the sensation of heartburn.

Avoiding the creation or aggravation of heartburn for your pregnant client should be taken into consideration when placing her on your massage table. The same type of positioning used to prevent Supine Hypotensive Syndrome will also prevent you from increasing her heartburn symptoms.

HEADACHES

Headaches are common in pregnancy especially in the first few months. Women who have never experienced any problems with headaches will complain.

Women who are prone to having headaches can have their problem intensify when pregnant. Again, the medical textbooks discuss different theories about why pregnant women have headaches, but there is no known reason. Any massage methods you use that are successful for the relief of headaches in nonpregnant clients would be appropriate to use on the pregnant client. Relaxation for tension headaches works well. Any technique you employ for the reduction of stress will be helpful.

A very effective nonchemical, noninvasive method of relieving headaches, especially migraine headaches, combines the use of hot and cold hydrotherapy. Place the headache sufferer in a comfortable sitting position. Prepare a foot bath with hot water at least 105 degrees Fahrenheit. Help her to gradually ease each part of her feet into the hot water since it will feel uncomfortably warm in the beginning. Place an ice pack at the base of her neck. Have her relax in this position for at least fifteen minutes. In my practice, I find the only barrier to the successful use of this method is that the person suffering from the headache (especially a migraine) is so uncomfortable from the pain and accompanying nausea, that she lacks the energy it takes to prepare the foot bath and ice pack. When teaching this technique, prepare the woman to engage the participation of family members in this type of treatment for headaches.

Those of you who employ such methods as shiatsu, acupressure, or reflexology for the relief of headache, I know of no harmful effects of these techniques on pregnancy. However, I offer the following observations.

Some textbooks dealing with reflexology, shiatsu, acupressure, and acupuncture have identified energy meridians around the area of the ankles, below the inner knee area, and the soft tissue between the thumb and forefinger as areas in which stimulation should be avoided when massaging pregnant clients. The books caution that stimulation of these areas can cause miscarriage or precipitate unwanted labor. (See Figure 20.)

There is no scientific data available to demonstrate that stimulation of any energy meridians does, indeed, create labor. The massage profession and the western obstetrical profession have not had the knowledge, resources, or desire to conduct controlled studies dealing with this subject. Except for the studies done by Dr. Dundee and Nurse-Midwife Hyde mentioned earlier, there is no quantitative data available that deals with acupressure and any aspect of pregnancy.

Any drugs for the relief of headaches in the pregnant woman should be prescribed by her medical caregiver.

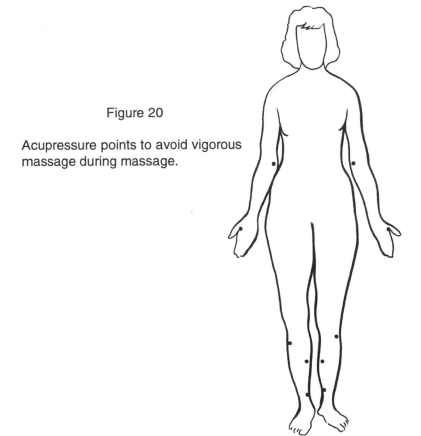

Figure 20

Acupressure points to avoid vigorous massage during massage.

BACKACHES (NONPATHOLOGICAL)

Nonpathological means pain or discomfort that is not caused by a disease process. The unique structure of the round ligament and the uterosacral ligament, that allows the uterus in pregnancy to rise from a pelvic organ to an abdominal organ, also contributes to low backache in pregnant women. The uterosacral ligament is a prominent band that extends in an upward curve from just above the cervix, along the lateral wall of the pelvis, and attaches deep within the faschia of the sacrum. The forward and downward pull of the uterus and its growing contents, increases the natural concave curve of the lower back creating constant muscle spasm.

The constant contraction of the lower back muscles results in relaxation of the other back supporting musculature, the abdominal muscles. This relaxation is further complicated by the extra stretching of the abdominal muscles by the enlarging uterus as it grows upward and outward. This can be even more of a problem if the woman failed to regain muscle tone of the abdominis recti muscles following prior pregnancies.

Massage techniques for the relief of back pain are part of the education of massage therapists. I am sure you have developed your own special methods of touch and treatment for backache in your nonpregnant clients. As long as you pay attention to the manner in which you position your pregnant clients on the table, avoiding the supine position, any massage modality that gives relief certainly would be appropriate.

Exercises to strengthen the supporting back muscles, such as the pelvic rock, may help with the relief of some low back pain. Teaching your client good body mechanics in lifting is certainly appropriate.

Good body mechanics for lifting should always be done from a bent-knee position rather than bending from the waist. Legs should be well spread and one foot should be placed slightly in front of the other. This gives a solid and broad base for balance when bending to lift. Pull the object close to the body before grasping, and rise allowing the leg muscles to do the lifting. (See Figure 21.)

A word about hot packs and the use of heat in pregnancy—it is considered dangerous to the fetus if the mother's core temperature rises above 104 degrees F. The core temperature of the body is defined as the inner temperature of the torso of the body and is usually 101 degrees F. Saunas, hot tubs, or tanning booths can raise the body's core temperature. To prevent this risk, hot packs applied to the back area of the pregnant woman should be monitored closely. Heat methods such as electric heating pads should never be applied. Heliotherapy or heat from infrared lamps should not be used.

Figure 21

Good body mechanics for lifting.

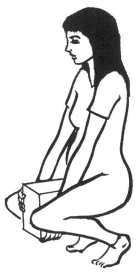

CARPAL TUNNEL SYNDROME

Most massage therapists have some knowledge about Carpal Tunnel Syndrome since it is an occupational hazard for massage therapist. The massage therapist may have symptoms because of overuse and strain of the hands and wrist in the course of repetitive daily use over time. The pregnant woman's symptoms are caused by the increased fluid volume created by the pregnancy. The average increase in blood volume during pregnancy is approximately 45 percent. However, in some women the blood volume will almost double. Most of this increase fluid volume stays in the circulatory system, but some is also held within the interstitial spaces. This can cause constant pressure and narrowing of the carpal tunnel space compressing the median nerve at the wrist. After delivery of her baby, the mother's blood volume returns to normal and the symptoms spontaneously disappear.

Typical symptoms are pain, numbness, or tingling in the thumb, one-half of the hand, or both hands, and is most commonly experienced upon awakening in the morning. *Williams Obstetrics* says as many as twenty-five percent of pregnant women will have some symptoms of this problem.

Many of the massage modalities address therapy for Carpal Tunnel Syndrome. Using whatever modality that has worked for you on nonpregnant patients certainly would not harm your client. However, the condition is caused by the pregnancy, thus, treating the symptoms rather than the condition is the more appropriate approach.

In the relaxed position the fingers gently curl in toward the palms. It is this natural curling toward the palm, pulling the ligaments during sleep, that places stress on the median nerve that is already compressed by the increase of fluids in the circulatory system creating the painful discomfort.

Splinting of the hand with the fingers straight for sleep usually gives immediate relief. A splint can be easily made using a one-inch Ace bandage and a piece of stiff cardboard. On the cardboard draw an outline of the palm and fingers leaving off the thumb portion on the cardboard. Cut out the cardboard outline, place it on the palm with the fingers extended straight out from the wrist, and wrap loosely with the one-inch Ace bandage. If your client's symptoms are in both hands, she can engage her partner or other family member in helping her with the splinting process.

Your client may find this splinting awkward, especially if she has symptoms in both extremities. However, she will find the relief she receives from the splinting well worth any awkwardness she may experience.

Chapter Three

MATERNAL PSYCHOLOGICAL ADJUSTMENT

Pregnancy is a time of change and transition for your pregnant client—change and transition between what her life was before she was pregnant and what her life will be like as the mother of the child she is carrying. It will be helpful to you if you understand that some of her emotional reactions are related, to some degree, to her biological changes or reactions to the hormones produced by the pregnancy.

This is a time in which she will be very open to her feelings and has a need to share this with others. If her spouse, significant other, or her family members are not willing to listen to her, you may find yourself in the role of listening to her talk about her feelings.

Be aware of this, and do not allow her sharing of her deep and private feelings to create anxiety for you. Another important aspect of this sharing is for you to understand that she is seeking an audience. She is not seeking advise. Do not offer advice. And remember that what she says to you is confidential.

Pregnancy is generally treated in the medical literature as a time of crisis progressing through somewhat predictable events that end with childbirth. For ease of understanding, these events can be broken down into three separate time frames: first, second and third trimesters. A trimester is a period of 3 months. The first trimester is the period of time from conception until the end of the 13th week of pregnancy. The second trimester is the period of gestation from week 14 and ends at the end of week 27. The third trimester begins at week 28 and ends at the birth of the baby.

FIRST TRIMESTER

To a large degree, the first trimester for the pregnant woman is a period of emotionally adjusting to the fact that she is pregnant. If completely honest with herself, she is upset and happy at the same time. Some of her emotions will include anxiety, disappointment, rejection, depression, and unhappiness along with the happiness of being pregnant. More than likely, she has said to herself that she did not want to be pregnant. This includes those women who have planned for and even struggled to become pregnant.

Along with all this she will feel guilty—guilty for having sad feelings. She may believe that a good mother should not experience negative feelings. She may think she is the only one who ever had these negative thoughts or feelings, and may hide these feelings, especially from her family. Her negative feelings usually end when she accepts the pregnancy, usually around the end of the first trimester

Most miscarriages take place in the first trimester of pregnancy, so this can be an anxious time of waiting for the pregnancy to be well established. This is particularly true for the woman who has had a previous miscarriage.

Her weight is also important at this time. Weight gain will be seen as proof of the pregnancy. If she sees her belly growing, it is physical confirmation, or proof, of the pregnancy.

On the other hand, a pregnant women who is trying to hide her pregnancy, such as an unwed teenager, may starve herself to prevent showing while trying to cope with and make decisions to resolve some of her problems.

Women will vary widely in their sexual desires in pregnancy beginning even in the first trimester. A woman's desire for sex can be reduced by fatigue, nausea, depression, sore and enlarged breasts, worries, anxieties, and concerns—all of which may be a normal part of her emotional adjustment to the pregnancy. Also, many women throughout pregnancy will have an increased need for love and loving without sex. Your pregnant client may choose you as an audience to air her anxieties surrounding this type of change. Reassuring the client of the normalcy of her feelings is appropriate. However, it is risky behavior to get into counseling about sexual problems.

If you follow the guidelines in the marketing chapter—not accepting a new massage client while still in her first trimester—it is possible you will not be involved in these first-trimester events. However, if an established client becomes pregnant and you continue your professional relationship as her massage therapist, it will be helpful to have knowledge of these first-trimester conflicts.

SECOND TRIMESTER

The second trimester, 14 though 27 weeks, is often referred to as the period of radiant health. During this period the pregnant woman's fatigue, nausea, breast tenderness, and other physical discomforts are gone. She feels good. She is free of the discomforts that will come later when she is large with child.

During the beginning of this trimester, she undergoes a complete reliving and re-evaluation of all aspects of her relationship with her mother. She will examine and analyze all the relationship problems she may have had with her mother. During this period, she comes to an understanding and acceptance of her mother's qualities that she values and respects. She will reject, as unwanted, the qualities of her mother that she does not value and respect. This rejection of parts of her mother may cause guilt as well as anxiety and conflict, unless she is able to reach the understanding that this process is normal and natural. It is not rejection of her mother. It is part of how she develops her own identity as a mother, how she adopts and adapts her mothering abilities.

Sometime around 20 weeks if this is her first pregnancy, a woman will begin to feel the baby moving. If she has had a successful pregnancy before, this awareness of the baby moving begins around 16 weeks. This is called quickening.

With quickening comes a number of changes. The pregnancy is verified. For the first time she may actually believe she is pregnant. She can see her baby as an individual and not just part of herself. This is the time when bonding with the baby begins. This is a time when she is most anxious for her partner to experience with her the realization of the baby as a person. She will have great curiosity and interest in the gender of the baby. She may even begin to refer to the baby as "she" or "he."

Her interests and activities will focus on pregnancy. As she goes about her usual activities, she will become more aware of pregnant women—pregnant women in stores, restaurants, places of entertainment, at work. Her social contacts increasingly become other pregnant women and new mothers. Her whole focus will be on pregnancy, childbearing, and preparation for the new role.

These types of changes create the need for a certain amount of grief work. This grief work involves letting go of former relationships and attachments that apply to both family and friends. She will no longer be the carefree friend who is available for last minute movies or meals out. Whether or not she agrees to it or feels she is ready, motherhood thrusts upon her the responsibilities of adulthood.

This letting go of significant aspects and events of her former self does not mean she discards all relationships and ties, but it does involve a change in, and toward, them. Also, this aspect is important for the woman who has other children. She will experience a certain disengagement from established ties with her other children as she prepares both the home and the family for the changes a new baby will bring. This is a fine line she walks, and it takes skill and energy to find her way along this necessary path.

THIRD TRIMESTER

The third trimester is the period from 28 weeks until delivery of the baby. It is often referred to as the period of watchful waiting. The woman grows impatient for the baby's arrival. The baby's movements become stronger with kicks that the mother can see as well as feel. The fetal movements and her increasing size are constant reminders of the baby.

A number of fears surface during this last trimester, especially fear of the unknown. She wonders if the baby will be healthy or not. She worries about labor, pain, and loss of control. She worries about whether or not she will know when she is in labor, and whether she will get to the hospital on time. She worries about the damage the pregnancy causes her body or vital organs. She worries about the loss of her youthful figure. She may even project adult emotions onto the baby evidenced by comments about the baby deliberately kicking her, or moving constantly at night to keep her awake.

This will be a time of intense dreaming for her, dreams about babies and children, and dreams about having the baby. She may have nightmares about the events surrounding the birth or nightmares of deformed babies. These intense dreams serve the purpose of helping her work through some of her fears and conflicts, and are considered healthy.

She will also experience another grief process as she anticipates the loss of attention and special status of being pregnant. This loss includes the separation of the baby from her body.

Because of her increased size and physical discomfort, she may feel awkward, ugly, sloppy, fat, and in need of large and frequent doses of reassurance from her mate.

Whatever she is experiencing—good and bad—know that your work with her as provider of therapeutic massage will be an important positive component of how she deals with the emotional changes associated with pregnancy. Again, you can help her as a good listener if she finds that confiding in you is safe.

Chapter Four

LABOR (GIVING BIRTH)

The word "labor" in the New Webster's Expanded Dictionary is defined as, "Exertion, physical or mental; toil; work done or to be done; the pangs and efforts of childbirth." The act of giving birth refers to a piece of work the body must do—labor. Athletes polled about working the body agree that when the body works for long periods, it creates pain. It will be helpful to your pregnant client if you can help her understand and adopt the concept that the labor of giving birth is a piece of work that the body performs. Giving birth is probably the hardest work most women will ever perform in our culture today and working the body creates pain.

Digging a ditch outdoors in the hot summer with a regular garden shovel for sixteen hours nonstop is hard work and creates pain. Ditch digging would be much easier and much less painful if a backhoe was used for the work of digging. With better tools the "piece of work" is easier. Today the woman does not have to do the work of giving birth alone. It is not a "bite-the-bullet" event. There are tools available to help make her work easier. Using these tools will help her perform the work of labor with less pain.

Tools for the performance of labor include: education about the labor process; having a labor coach or support person(s) present; pain medications; nurses, midwives, and physicians; having a controlled and safe environment; and TOUCH.

This is the concept that supports your role in helping your pregnant client carry out the work of labor. You are one of the tools that can help her do the hard work of giving birth. You have been performing massage during the prenatal period. You have a good knowledge of what type of touch she is comfortable with. You are able to recognize her tension. You know what depth of massage she can tolerate. You are the expert in touch. In order to be effective in your role as support person (Doula) for the laboring woman, you must, to some degree, become expert in the process of labor.

Throughout the pregnancy she has been having Braxton Hicks contractions especially in the latter months. Braxton Hicks contractions are a tightening of the uterus, usually painless, lasting from several seconds to several minutes. They are irregular in pattern. The purpose of Braxton Hicks contractions is nature's way or training or preparing the uterus for its marathon athletic event of giving birth.

Braxton Hicks contractions can create confusion in the diagnosis of labor. The massage therapist should not attempt to determine the character of contractions or advise the pregnant client about contractions, especially before she has completed 36 weeks of gestation. Any questions or problems your pregnant client has about contractions need to be referred to her midwife or physician.

The end of the pregnancy can be a period of what Varney, in her book *Midwifery*, refers to as "the miseries at the end of the pregnancy." The pregnant woman will have muscular aches and pains; low back pain; pain in the abdomen; leg cramps. She will be tired of being pregnant, tired of feeling large and clumsy. She may be upset and angry because labor has not started. She may not be able to rest or sleep. If she has other children to care for, resting during the daytime hours will be impossible unless she has family or friends she can call on.

All the skills of the massage therapist can be utilized to help her deal with these miseries. The relaxation and stress reduction techniques for the relief of aches and pain, and the nurturing touch in the hour on your massage table can give her relief that lasts for hours and days.

The exact triggers for labor have not been discovered. There is probably not a single trigger involved, but a series of triggers, physical and chemical, that work similar to dominoes, one activating the next. The change from the uterus holding the fetus inside, to its decision to force the fetus out, includes the production of hormones. It is also theorized that a decrease in the production of certain hormones is part of the trigger pattern. However, there remains many unanswered questions about how labor starts.

Williams Obstetrics defines labor as a physiological and clinical event and divides it into three phases. Phase one: the time of uterine preparedness for labor is the period when the cervix loses its mucous plug and begins to soften and move from a posterior position in the back of the vagina to anterior or frontal position in the vagina. Phase two: the onset of labor or the time of forceful contractions by the uterus that opens the cervix, pushing the baby down and out the birth canal and subsequent delivery of the placenta. Phase three: the persistent contraction of the uterus to control bleeding and the following weeks in which the uterus returns to its nonpregnant status and size.

FIRST STAGE

Prodromal or early labor—1 to 3 centimeters dilation

The most important part of your expertise is not the medical description of labor, but labor as experienced by your pregnant client. Your client's labor experience usually begins with her awareness of the loss of her mucous plug. Hormones produced in these last weeks of the pregnancy change the cervix from a rigid consistency, similar to the pad of the thumb, to a soft mushy consistency. At the same time, the tenacious mucous that has filled and sealed the cervix from the beginning of the pregnancy will begin to break loose, creating a mucousy vaginal discharge. This mucous sometimes is tinged with pink or red streaks of blood. This is the event she has been waiting for, visible proof that labor is near.

Labor at term—after the completion of 36-weeks gestation—usually begins as a feeling of menstrual cramps or pain in the lower abdomen and can radiate to the low back. In some women the cramps begin in the low back and radiate to the lower abdomen. Along with the sensation of cramping pain, the woman will feel her abdomen tighten and become soft in a regular pattern. Some women start labor contractions right away, 5 minutes apart, but most women will begin the regular pattern of labor contractions 15 to 20 minutes apart. As time passes they become closer together and stronger in intensity. Early labor contractions last only a few seconds—20 to 30 seconds. As the labor contractions grow stronger they last longer—45 to 60 seconds. It is common for the pregnant woman to have some diarrhea. She may have a pink or red tinged vaginal discharge. She may rupture or break her bag of water. Rupture of the bag of water can be a large gush of fluid, or it can be a small leak. Any fluid coming from the vagina means it is time to leave for the birthing center or hospital.

During this early phase of labor she will be excited and anxious at the same time. She will want to contact the people who plan to be with her during the labor. She will want her spouse/significant other present. She will be tempted to leave for the birthing site now.

If she is a first-time mother, her medical caregiver has instructed her to wait until her contractions are 5 minutes apart. If she has had a baby before, her medical caregiver will have instructed her to plan to leave home for the birthing center/hospital when her contractions are 8 to 10 minutes apart. Instructions will vary based on the policies of where she plans to deliver and the distance to the birthing site.

ROLE OF MASSAGE THERAPIST AS DOULA

1. Encourage the woman during this period to complete any last minute arrangements.

2. This is a time for her to consider getting as much rest as possible, practice relaxation techniques, soak in a warm tub, or take a warm shower and shampoo.

3. It is too early for her to begin breathing techniques.

4. If hungry, she can eat light snacks that are easy to digest. During the active labor phase, digestion slows down.

5. The contractions become stronger and harder. She is comfortable between the contractions, smiling, excited, talkative, asking questions, and sharing her symptoms. As the contractions become stronger and harder, she is having to stop to breathe and is unable to talk. It is time to go to the birthing site (birthing center/hospital).

Active Phase of First Stage—4 to 10 centimeters dilation

The pregnant woman will have an evaluation by her medical provider and will be admitted officially as a patient. Walking stimulates true labor and eases false labor. This is the time for walking. She will be more comfortable if she is encouraged to walk and labor will progress faster than if she is placed in bed.

First-time mothers may be surprised and overwhelmed by contractions that are more painful than imagined. Dry mouth after breathing through the contraction is common. She will be perspiring. She may experience nausea or vomiting. She may become more and more uncomfortable and annoyed with the contractions.

In normal labor, a first-time mother will dilate approximately 1 centimeter an hour. If she has had a baby before, she will dilate more than 1 centimeter an hour. As she labors and time passes, she may become tired. She will be less able to relax and less able to cope. She may become anxious and moan and cry out.

ROLE OF THERAPIST AS DOULA
IN ACTIVE PHASE

1. Use ice massage during the contractions if she finds this gives her relief. (See technique for ice massage at the end of this chapter.)

2. Check for relaxation during the contractions. Help her with relaxation with verbal cues and with touch. Rub her feet, hands, scalp, any other place that she finds soothing and relaxing. This is the time for maximizing touch. Later on she may not be able to tolerate being touched.

3. Check her breathing during the contractions. Help her with her technique if necessary.

4. Listen to her. Praise her efforts. Stay close to her whether she is up walking or lying in bed.

5. Try position changes if in bed. Encourage her to urinate frequently.

6. If medical facility policy allows, encourage sips of liquids or ice chips. Offer lip gloss or balm.

7. Offer cool damp cloth to head. Fan her if she is hot.

8. If available, encourage her to get into whirlpool bath or shower.

9. If it helps, encourage her to make noises along with the breathing during contractions.

10. Stay close to her and make lots of eye-to-eye contact.

As she approaches the end of the dilating phase, 7 to 10 centimeters, she will be working very hard. The contractions are now 1 to 3 minutes apart and lasting 60 to 90 seconds, peaking early, and sometimes with the urge to push. She may have nausea or vomiting, shaking of her upper thighs, and cramping in her hips, thighs, or legs. Her bag of water may break. This may frighten her. She may find she is less and less able to cope with the pain and intensity of the contractions. She will be totally focused on herself and will want constant companionship.

If she has the desire to push before she is completely dilated, encourage her to grunt with a growling sound deep in her throat during the contraction. This allows for gentle pushing without tiring her more and helps her cope with her body's urge to push prematurely.

SECOND STAGE—PUSHING

Many times when the pregnant woman reaches 10 centimeters she will have the urge to push, but the contractions may slow down, giving her a chance to rest. She will be re-energized, awake, and alert. The urge to push will be strong and her body will involuntarily push or bear down. Pushing will be a relief from the intense pain of the contractions.

Position for pushing can be done on either right or left side or in an upright position. Let her choose which feels best. Whatever position she chooses, help her to grasp her knees or behind her knees and pull toward her shoulders with the knees outward to open up the hip area while pushing. Her chin should rest on her chest, curling her spine into a "C" position. This directs the force of the pushing effort in the most effective direction.

This may be a time when she panics. She may suddenly be afraid and say that she "can't do it." She may decide she is going to simply quit and go home.

ROLE OF THE THERAPIST AS DOULA
IN SECOND STAGE

1. Help her assume whatever position is comfortable for pushing. Ice massage will not be helpful at this stage.

2. Hold her hands or help her grasp her legs or knees to give her leverage for pushing.

3. Extend and massage her legs if she has leg cramps after pushing.

4. Let her medical caregiver or nurse guide her in her pushing. Tell her in between pushing that she is pushing fine.

5. Tell her of the progress she is making, the bulging of the rectum, the flattening of the perineum, crowning of the baby's head.

6. Arrange for her to see her progress in a mirror, especially when she begins to crown.

7. Pushing is hard work. She will be sweating and hot. Arrange for someone to fan her. Use cool clothes to wipe her face, neck, hands, and any part of her body where she says it feels good.

As the head slowly emerges the medical caregiver directs her in pushing for delivery of the rest of the baby. The baby is usually placed on the mother's abdomen either before or after the cord is clamped and cut.

The mother and father will be engrossed in the baby, touching and looking and examining. The medical caregiver will deliver the placenta and make any suturing repairs needed. No matter how tired or exhausted during the labor process, the new mother will be alert, happy, joyful, talking, laughing, crying, and asking for reassurances about the baby. She may be apologetic about her behavior during labor.

Birth is also a spiritual experience for the mother and the father. Recognize this and support the spirituality of this event by helping to keep the environment nonintrusive. The work of mothering the mother during labor is done.

ICE MASSAGE FOR THE CONTROL OF LABOR PAIN

Ice massage for the control of labor pain is based on the work done by Dr. Ronald Melzack and Dr. Patrick Wall at the McGill University in Canada. In the early 1960s Drs. Melzack and Wall proposed a new theory of pain mechanism. According to their gate control theory of pain, stimulation of the skin creates nerve impulses that are transmitted to the spinal cord system. These nerve impulses can be inhibited or enhanced at the level of the spinal cord. Nerve impulses traveling toward the brain in the smaller nerve fibers of the spinal cord proceed at a steady rate. This continuous discharge keeps the pain gate open and the transmission of pain is enhanced. Nerve impulses traveling toward the brain through large nerve fibers in the spinal cord occur in a burst of impulses. These burst-type impulses are mainly inhibitory and have the effect of keeping the pain gate partially closed resulting in diminishing pain intensity. When the large fiber impulses are artificially stimulated by vibration, scratching, or "ice massage" the gate further closes resulting in a decrease in the sensation of pain.

Ice has been successfully used in the treatment of musculoskeletal pain over the years. Dr. Melzack studied the use of ice massage of the web of skin between the thumb and forefinger for the reduction of acute dental pain. His work showed a 50 percent reduction of acute dental pain. Having experienced both dental and childbirth pain, I felt that the intensity of the two were comparable. If ice massage of the web of skin between the thumb and forefinger could reduce dental pain, it could also reduce labor pain.

A search of the literature revealed Aleda Erskin, et al., in 1990 published a literature review about memory of pain. Under the category of "acute clinical pain" she linked dental and childbirth pain. This was scientific data supporting my empirical data—the intensity of the two types of pain were comparable.

Back to the library and the literature about pain, I found that Dr. Melzack and Dr. W. S. Torgenson had developed a tool for the measurement of pain called the McGill Pain

Questionnaire. This tool has been tested for consistent results and has stood the test of time within scientific circles. With the measurement tool in hand, a protocol for choosing laboring women was developed.

The application of ice massage to the skin is noninvasive, nonpharmaceutical, and is comparable to applying a hot water bottle or powder for effleurage and is no threat to the mother or the fetus. A study of the use of ice massage for the control of labor pain over a six-month period was carried out in 1992.

Results of the Study

Eighty-six percent of the women in the study experienced a decrease in pain unpleasantness as well as a decrease in pain intensity. The following table shows how the study members dropped in rank in describing their memory of pain unpleasantness. (See Table 1.)

The study was designed to carry out ice massage of the web of skin between the thumb and forefinger for a period of thirty minutes, however, fifty-seven percent of the women in the study felt they received so much relief as a result of the intervention with the ice that they continued with the ice massage, requesting family and nurses to perform the ice massage until the end of the first stage of labor. Some participants felt they had more relief on one hand than the other.

Additional findings from the study indicate that the use of ice massage results in some women dilating much faster than the rate predicted by a standard labor curve (1 centimeter per hour more or less depending on how many times the laboring woman had been pregnant).

Located within the anatomical area used for ice massage is an acupressure meridian referred to as Large Intestine 4 or LI4. Acupressure literature identifies LI4 as a point to be avoided before time for labor to begin. However, during labor, stimulation of LI4 is recommended to speed up labor.

PAIN LEVEL	BEFORE ICE	AFTER ICE
Excruciating	21.4%	7.1%
Horrible	42.9%	21.4%
Distressing	7.1%	14.3%
Mild	0.0%	14.3%

Table 1

How-to, hands-on ice massage for the control of labor pain

1. Tools needed are: Crushed ice and a small washcloth.

2. Place a small amount of crushed ice in the center of the washcloth. Twist the washcloth around the ice making a miniature ice bag.

3. At the beginning of each contraction use the ice bag to massage the web of skin between the thumb and forefinger continuously until the end of the contraction. (See Figure 22.)

4. The pressure of the massage should measure about a 6 on a scale of 1 being very light pressure and 10 being pressure as hard as you can apply.

5. Experiment with massage on each hand to find which hand works best.

6. Some women—thirteen percent in my study—will find that ice massage does not reduce labor pain. If the woman feels it does not help, stop.

7. It is not practical to attempt to continue ice massage once she reaches the pushing stage. Plus, the act of pushing relieves pain.

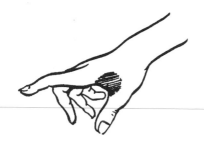

Figure 22

Anatomical location for ice massage during labor contraction.

NOTE:

Ice massage for the control of labor pain, a research project, was carried out at Dade City Hospital, Dade City, Florida, in 1992. The study was presented as a research paper at University of Southern Queensland, Toowoomba, Queensland, Australia, June 1992 and at a Midwifery Education Seminar at Tampa General Hospital, Tampa, Florida, 1993.

CHAPTER FIVE

MASSAGE THERAPIST AS DOULA

Your prenatal client will view the labor and birth as the major experience of her pregnancy. All of the events of the past nine months, good or bad, unpleasant or joyful, pale in comparison to how she anticipates and prepares for the actual labor and birth. As she approaches this time, she can have many emotions, ranging from great relief that the event is beginning, to panic and fear of the process of labor. Your prenatal client may have doubts about what kind of mother she will be. She might be reluctant to give up her pregnant role and the attention she gained during the pregnancy. Whatever her emotional or mental state when beginning the labor process, successful completion of the labor and birth empowers her in a broad sense of her womanhood, her femininity, and her strength. I remember a young teen client of mine with a childhood history of abuse and poor mothering. At the time her labor began, she progressed so rapidly through the labor there was no time to administer any type of pain medications. Six hours after her noisy, fast and normal delivery, she was walking around the birthing room drying her hair after a shower—muttering at first—"I did natural childbirth." She proceeded to laughing and hugging herself, twirling in a dance and shouting, "I did natural childbirth."

When your pregnant client goes to the hospital or birthing center to give birth, she will have family members present. When needed, she will have nurses, a midwife, or a physician. However, unless your client delivers in a birthing center, she will not have continuous, one-to-one professional support from nursing staff, midwife, or physician. If she delivers in a hospital, her labor more than likely will include intravenous infusions. She will not be allowed to eat. She may receive injections of medication that facilitate labor and reduce pain. She may not be allowed out of bed to walk. Continuous electronic monitoring of her labor contractions and the unborn baby may be carried out. Many of these interventions interfere with the natural course of labor resulting in the need for delivery with vacuum extractors, forceps, or surgical delivery by cesarean.

Women who have attended childbirth education classes will have a labor coach, usually the father of the baby. Sometimes the labor coach will be her mother, sister, or friend. Her labor coach will have had childbirth classes along with the new mother. But many times her labor coach, especially the husband or significant other, may be poorly prepared for the events of real labor—length of the labor (some can last for 24 to 36 hours or more); odors; sight of blood, vomit, feces; and feelings of helplessness at witnessing a loved one in pain. If the mother is the caretaker in her relationship with the labor coach, the coach may be unable to nurture her, and may also be experiencing a need for nurturing.

As her massage therapist during the pregnancy, you have decreased her stress, her pains and discomforts with touch and massage. You have been a listener. You know about her family and her circumstances. You have given her appropriate education and reassurance. Who better able to serve as a professional support person in labor, or DOULA, than you, her massage therapist?

WHAT IS A DOULA?

Doula is a Greek word meaning "in service of," and historically has been an older experienced woman who is present during labor to support and guide the new mother through the labor, and later, teach and support her in caring for her new baby. The word doula first appeared in the medical journals in the United States in a scientific study reported in the *New England Journal of Medicine,* September 11, 1980. This study was done by Drs. John Kennell and Marshall Klaus, et al. The initial study was conducted at the Social Security Hospital, Guatemala City, Guatemala, and later repeated at Jefferson Davis Hospital in Houston, Texas. The second study was published in the *Journal of The American Medical Association,* May 1, 1991.

Since 1980, the word doula has been adopted by the natural childbirth movement. Articles describing the doula have appeared in publications such as *Birthing* and *Midwifery Today,* and more recently in mainstream publications such as *Science News, Newsweek, Parenting Magazine,* and *American Baby.*

During this time the role of the doula has been expanded from the labor support duties first described by Drs. Kennell and Klaus, to encompass in-home postpartum services. These services include nurturing, or mothering the mother, infant care instructions and assistance, and light housework.

A massage therapist in private practice or as an employee of a massage facility may not have the time or may not choose to serve as doula during the postpartum period. However, the postpartum period is the time to continue regular massaging of the mother, nurturing of the mother, and offering infant massage instruction to both parents. (See chapters on postpartum period and infant massage.)

How can the massage therapist prepare for the role of doula during labor and birth? There is a how-to book entitled *Special Women, The Role Of The Professional Labor Assistant* by Paulina Perez and Cheryl Snedeker, published by Pennypress, Seattle, Washington, in 1990.

Lamaze Parents' Magazine contains a wealth of information about pregnancy, birth, the newborn, and the postpartum period. *Lamaze Parents' Magazine,* published by ASPO/ Lamaze, is distributed to expectant parents in childbirth classes and health care professionals, such as yourself, can receive free copies by calling 1-800-832-027 or writing:

Lamaze Publishing Company, Inc.
372 Danbury Road
Wilton, Connecticut 06897

There are few formal education courses offered. This will change as the doula movement is embraced by massage therapists who see the value of adding the specialty of prenatal massage to their practice

The Seattle Midwifery School, Extension Education Program, offers a two-fold curriculum for: 1) the education of labor support doulas, and 2) the preparation of doula trainers as faculty. These programs were developed by Penny Simkin, PT, a longtime pioneer in the work of natural childbirth and alternatives to high-tech obstetrics. These courses are offered on a regular basis in the Pacific Northwest and occasionally in other parts of the country. The address for information about their doula education program is:

Seattle Midwifery School
Extension Education
2524 16th Avenue, S. #300
Seattle, Washington 98144

You may also use this address to obtain information regarding the Pacific Association of Labor Support (PALS) and Doulas of North America (DONA).

If you are unable to attend a formal education course, there are some things I would recommend for massage therapists who wish to prepare for the labor support doula role.

1. Attend a formal childbirth education program—Lamaze, Bradley, etc. In this class you will learn relaxation and breathing techniques and how the couple is taught to practice at home. You will learn about pain relief in childbirth and the different methods of managing it. You will learn about birthing positions and how using a variety of positions can provide increased comfort. You will gain information on how to provide comfort and support to the mother. Having a step-by-step planning guide (birth plan) is a valuable tool and part of mastering natural childbirth skills. Most childbirth educators furnish class participants with a detailed, illustrated guide to the complete labor process. This guide provides information about typical changes in the laboring woman, gives helpful responses for the support person, and provides a description of the role of the medical care personnel (nurses, midwives, and physician).

2. Contact your local hospital and your local birthing centers. Ask for a tour of the facility and ask questions during the tour. Get to know the staff. If the hospital offers childbirth education classes, attend them. Hospital sponsored classes many times teach couples what to expect in the labor and delivery process at their particular facility, rather than the classical Lamaze preparation for childbirth. This is an excellent way to learn about available options in labor. Solicit the support of the these educators by sharing with them your planned role in your clients' use of their facility.

3. Complete the reading list for labor support doulas in Appendix 1 at the end of this book.

4. Become completely familiar with the stages and events of labor.

5. Add all the comfort measures gained from your education and experience as a massage therapist to your bag of tools for use at the labor event. In the laboring woman they work even better.

6. Offer labor support services free to any pregnant customer you may currently have in your caseload. This will give the opportunity for invaluable hands-on experience.

Remember, in the studies done by Drs. Kennel and Klaus, the doulas were laywomen with no formal medical or nursing education or experience. They were recruited and taught in a three-week course, to act as labor support persons. They were not educated in what we call, "Lamaze childbirth techniques." Their role was to stay with the laboring woman, whether she was in bed or walking. They had knowledge of the labor process and were able to explain to the laboring woman what was happening, answer her questions, and give her encouragement and reassurance. But most importantly, they touched the laboring woman. They stroked her. They made sure she was warm when needed. They helped her stay cool while she was doing the hard work of labor. They wiped her sweaty brow and face and hair with cool cloths. They rubbed her tired feet. They did abdominal effleurage and rubbed aching backs. And most importantly they TOUCHED. Who is the touch expert? The massage therapist. Again, who better to serve as labor support doula? The massage therapist.

CHAPTER SIX

THE POSTPARTUM PERIOD

The postpartum period is sometimes referred to as the fourth trimester, or the last quarter of the pregnant year. This infers that somehow we can make three (tri) into four. Technically, the postpartum time frame includes the six weeks immediately following the birth event. It is also referred to as the puerperium, meaning the period of confinement after childbirth. Modern medicine defines this period of time as the length of time it takes for the uterus, cervix, and vagina to return to their normal nonpregnant state.

THE POSTPARTUM UTERUS

Immediately after birth the uterus is about the size of a large grapefruit and weighs approximately 2 to 2½ pounds. It is not exactly round, but appears more like an inverted pear shape, larger at the top and smaller at the bottom. It will be located about midway between the umbilicus and the symphysis pubis or higher depending on how much urine is in the woman's bladder. Within 2 days after delivery, it will begin to shrink in size, weighing about 1 pound a week after delivery. At the end of the 2nd week it weighs about ¾ quarters pound and has descended back into the pelvic cavity. Within another week or so it becomes close to its original size. As in its growth process, the shrinking uterus is not a result of a decrease in the number of muscle cells, but a decrease in the size of the cells. It retains its ability to contract, but rids itself of most of the contractile proteins from the cells themselves.

Bleeding after giving birth is a result of large open blood vessels at the site of the attachment of the placenta. The placental site within the uterus immediately after the birth is about the size of the palm. Along with the shrinking size of the uterus, the placental site shrinks, becoming 3 to 4 centimeters by the end of 2 weeks, completely disappearing at the end of 6 weeks. The miracle of this repairing process within the uterus is that there is no scar left on the uterine wall. Growth of underlying tissue completely erases any evidence of placental implantation, leaving the entire uterine lining smooth and without scars, ready to receive placental implantation from future pregnancies.

Other physiologic changes include a return to normal of the renal system, the gastrointestinal system, and blood pressure. The birth itself is equivalent to a super-crash diet, with the woman losing 12 pounds or more at the time of birth and another 5 pounds in the next week as the increased blood volume returns to normal.

The most immediate visible event surrounding the postpartum period for the woman is the return of her nonpregnant silhouette. She can again see her feet. She can move and bend with an ease she has not experienced in the past several months. If she has gained extra weight during the pregnancy, she will be concerned about her weight.

If she has stretch marks (striae), they will fade from red visible marks to silvery colored marks. By the end of 2 or 3 months she will have to search to find them. The pigmented line (linea nigra) down the center of her abdomen will fade during this time, as will any face discolorations (chloasma).

The wall of the abdomen is flabby after delivery as a result of the stretching of the abdominis recti muscles during the pregnancy. All women will have some degree of separation of the recti muscles of the abdomen. This condition is called diastasis recti. Diastasis means separation. It will be important for a woman to identify diastasis recti and take steps to regain closure and good muscle tone. Unless she is cared for by a midwife, it is likely the separation (diastasis) of the muscles will not be shown to her, nor will she have specific instructions on how to close the separation and regain her abdominal muscle tone. (See Figure 10.)

The massage therapist can play an important role in helping the postpartum woman identify any diastasis recti and motivate her to do the exercises required to restore the muscles to their prepregnancy state. In my practice I find that showing the woman the separation and telling her that if she does not fill the hole with muscle, it will fill up with fat is a strong motivator to do the work it takes for resolution. Truthfully, if the muscle tone of the abdominal wall muscles is not regained, the diastasis space fills with peritoneum membrane, faschia, and fat tissue.

HOW DO YOU CHECK FOR DIASTASIS RECTI?

Diastasis is the degree or amount of the separation of the abdominis recti muscles. Measure this separation in fingerbreadths by asking the woman to contract her muscles in the following manner:

1. Have her lie in a supine position on the massage table. Hands are cupped under her head. Knees are bent with feet flat on the table and knees hip-width apart.

2. Standing at her side, place the tips of your fingers over the midline of her abdomen at the level of the umbilicus (navel). Ask her to raise her head and shoulders toward her

chest, keeping her elbows pointed outward. This will iso-
late and contract the abdominis recti muscles.

3. As the woman raises her head, press your fingers gently into
the abdomen. Feel the abdominal muscles like rubber bands
along each side of the midline of the abdomen. The space
between these muscle bands is measured in fingerbreadths.
She can have a separation space anywhere from 1 to 5
fingerbreadths.

4. It will be important for you to show her this separation. To
do so, grasp one of her hands and place her fingertips in
the same position you placed yours and again ask her to
raise her head and shoulders, allowing her to feel the separation.

5. She will probably be surprised at what you are showing her.
Explain to her how the muscles normally attach at the rib
cage, cover the abdomen, and connect in the symphysis
pubic area. As the uterus grows and rises up into the abdomen, the muscles stretch and separate creating this problem.

HOW TO REGAIN MUSCLE TONE IN THE ABDOMINIS RECTI

Explain how the abdominal muscles support the back and
how poor muscle tone can cause backaches. Poor muscle tone
can affect future pregnancies by causing abnormal presentations
at birth, such as buttocks first instead of head first (breech). In
my experience a woman's desire to regain her former physical
appearance—her figure—will be one of her strongest motiva-
tors to do the exercises required to resolve the diastasis. Do not
hesitate to use this.

Share with her the exercise you plan to teach her will also help her to rid herself of her "jelly belly."

The exercise to regain muscle tone in the abdominis recti is the same modified sit-up you asked her to perform on your table in order to check for the separation. Have her repeat the modified sit-up and show her how this exercise isolates and uses only the abdominis recti muscles. This exercise may be difficult for her if she has delivered in the last week or so. Trembling of her muscles during the demonstration or difficulty lifting her head and shoulders is evidence of poor muscle tone. If this occurs, use it to demonstrate the need to regain her strength in this muscle group.

She should repeat this exercise regimen daily until she cannot feel the separation. This may take five or six weeks. Of all the exercises that she may choose to perform in the post partum period, I feel this is the most important one for her to practice.

If she performs this exercise a minimum of ten times, three times a day, she will strengthen her abdominis recti, close the separation, and rid herself of any flabby tissue in her belly. (See Figure 23.)

Figure 23

Modified sit-up (crunches) to tone abdominis recti after the birth and close diastasis.

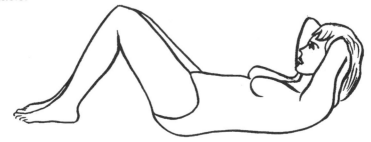

What other problems do you need to be concerned about during the postpartum period?

All women will have a discharge from the vagina after giving birth. The first 2 to 3 days the discharge consists almost entirely of blood from the large open vessels of the wall of the uterus where the placenta was attached. The amount varies, but in most women it is like having a heavy menstrual period. As the placental site begins to heal, the discharge changes to a paler color and the amount is decreased. Ten to 12 days postpartum the discharge changes to a yellow-white discharge and decreases to nothing in the next week or so.

During this period of time the massage therapist makes the postpartum woman feel comfortable with disrobing by providing generous draping and large disposable sanitary pads for use if needed.

Today over sixty percent of new mothers elect to breast feed their new babies. If your client is breast feeding (lactating), her breasts may be large and pendulous because they are filled with milk. Removal of her bra may result in some discomfort. A selection of small soft pillows to use for breast support in the different positions while on the table can contribute to her comfort and relaxation.

The nonlactating new mother may experience some of the same discomforts when removing her bra especially in the first couple of weeks postpartum. Even though she has chosen not to breast feed, her breasts will make milk. Any extra stimulation of the breasts in this early postpartum period is contraindicated because it increases milk production. Particular care should be made to offer her pillows for support and comfort while on your table and to avoid any tactile stimulation of the breasts.

Are there any absolute contraindications to massage in the postpartum period?

Yes. A postpartum condition known as deep venous thrombosis or blood clots in the leg was fairly frequent as late as the 1950s when it was common practice to keep the new mother from getting out of bed and walking for up to a week after the birth. The condition was commonly called "milk leg." In more recent years there has been a major decrease in the frequency of this condition. However, *Williams Obstetrics* states pregnant or postpartum women have an increased incidence when compared to nonpregnant women of similar age.

The symptoms of deep venous thrombosis are an abrupt onset of severe pain and edema, and heat and redness of the leg and thigh. Usually this condition involves most of the deep venous system from the foot to the iliofemoral region.

Massage, especially deep tissue massage, in a client with any degree of deep venous thrombosis, can serve to dislodge small blood clots that can travel to the lungs becoming a life-threatening event.

Because some women can have a dangerous amount of deep vein clots with little reaction in the way of heat, pain, or swelling, a simple easy assessment of both extremities should be carried out on all your postpartum clients. In the supine position with legs straight, using both hands on each side of the client's leg, palpate each extremity for tenderness and abnormal heat. Next stretch the Achilles tendon on both extremities (Homan's sign) by placing the leg straight on your table. Apply gentle pressure on the knee, keeping the leg straight. With the other hand, firmly flex the foot toward her chin. (See Figure 16.)

The sign is positive if this maneuver creates any pain in the leg. A positive Homan's sign could be due to benign conditions such as muscle strain or a bruise. However, in the presence of tenderness, abnormal heat, or a positive Homan's sign, massage should be postponed and the client referred to her medical provider for evaluation. Prudent massage therapists will make Homan's sign testing and documentation a regular part of assessment before beginning a massage on a pregnant or postpartum client.

POSTPARTUM EMOTIONAL REACTION

In addition to resolution of physical changes during the pregnancy, the postpartum period is a time of emotional changes. Beginning on the 3rd to 5th day after the birth the mother will be sensitive, get upset easily, feel sad, and even cry for seemingly no reason. She may not be able to explain why she is crying. Medical terminology used to describe these symptoms is postpartum depression or "postpartum blues."

Postpartum blues is a self-limiting event usually disappearing after the second week and is fairly common. Thus, it is thought to be a "normal" reaction to childbirth and not looked at seriously by the medical community.

My own personal feeling about postpartum blues is that seventy-five percent of symptoms are a direct result of fatigue. Normally a woman feels physically well after childbirth. Because she feels well physically, she is tempted to immediately return to the management of her normal household duties. She may feel guilty and unworthy of "being taken care of" and assume household work even when she does not feel up to it.

Within the uterus is an open wound where the placenta was attached. This open wound is why she bleeds after childbirth. If new mothers were sent home with an incision in the belly with sutures or staples, an acute awareness that her body was healing and rest was required would dictate her daily routine.

Under the very best of conditions during the postpartum period, the mother will not have more than two or three hours of unbroken sleep for the next few months. For the breast feeding mother sleep periods can be less.

The woman will also face the task of grieving about the loss of her pregnant state. She has lost her "star" status. Family and friends will have shifted their attention to the new baby. This shift can result in the loss of nurturing the postpartum woman needs as she assumes the role and responsibilities of being a mother. It is well established in the medical literature that the key to good mothering is for the mother to receive nurturing.

If the couple does not live close to family members who are part of their supportive network, the burden of emotional support falls upon the husband or significant other. He may be overwhelmed by his experience of the birth event and his work of assuming the role of father. Today's practice of sending mothers and babies home from the hospital twenty-four hours after birth, with all the physical demands and adjustments a new baby can create, places a huge amount of extra stress on the mother and the father.

Continuation of massage during the postpartum period is an important tool for dealing with postpartum blues. It offers a rest from the responsibilities of caring for a new baby. It gives important nurturing to the mother, impacting in a highly positive manner her ability to mother. Note: supine position is safe for massage in the postpartum period.

CHAPTER SEVEN

INFANT MASSAGE

"We must gorge them with warmth and caresses just as we do with milk," says Frederick Leboyer, M.D. in *Loving Hands*. Without touch babies die, thus, touching and massaging of babies is as old as the human race.

The purpose of devoting a chapter on infant massage is not specifically to teach infant massage, but to share some of the scientific studies about massage and infants; to look at the history of the infant massage education movement; to examine some important anatomy and physiology associated with infant massage; and hopefully to give you the confidence to add infant massage teaching to the services you offer the pregnant woman and her family.

HISTORY OF INFANT MASSAGE IN THE UNITED STATES

One of the first books about infant massage to catch the attention of American parents was *Loving Hands, The Traditional Indian Art of Baby Massage*, by Fredrick Leboyer, M.D., an obstetrician from France. Some of its popularity was probably associated with the success of Dr. Leboyer's first book, *Birth Without Violence* (1973), in which he describes his work in France with gentle birth. He writes about gentle, quiet, loving, and nurturing environments at the time of birth. His work helped change obstetrics as it was practiced in this country. Dr. Leboyer's book about infant massage is more a beautiful work of art rather than a how-to book for massage. It has superb black and white photos of women in India massaging their babies and the text is more poetry than prose.

The Baby Massage Book, a how-to book, by Tina Heinl, published in 1982, describes how she was given a present of Dr. Leboyer's book, *Loving Hands,* and used his book to develop her infant massage techniques which she practiced on her children. Heinl produced a beautiful book with watercolor illustrations of all the infant massage positions and massage strokes. She includes the Indian method of squeezing, twisting, and stroking from the shoulder to the hand and from the thigh to the foot, pushing blood against the normal flow of the bloodstream.

Baby Massage, another how-to book, by Amelia Auckett, published in Australia in 1981 and later distributed in the United States, advocates using the techniques shown in Dr. Leboyer's book—squeezing, twisting, and stroking the arms and legs against the natural flow of the bloodstream.

Infant Massage, A Handbook for Loving Parents, by Vimala Schneider McClure, is probably the most well-known how-to book. McClure bases her infant massage techniques on her experiences while studying and working in India and describes the Indian milking technique which is squeezing, twisting, and stroking of the extremities that pushes blood against the normal blood flow current.

Along with her massage program, McClure founded the International Association of Infant Massage Instructors. The I.A.I.M.I. educates teachers of infant massage and teaches parents infant massage techniques.

One of the best descriptions of infant massage, why and how its importance impacts on parent-infant bonding and infant development, appears in *Advances in Touch, New Implications in Human Development,* published by Johnson & Johnson.

The description is written by Laurie Evans, M.A., instructor trainer, International Association of Infant Massage Instructors. Evans describes the grassroots instructor education program. She goes on to explain how massage of the infant is not only a major tool to soothe the baby with tactile stimulation, but is also a major loving and verbal communication tool.

SCIENTIFIC STUDIES ABOUT MASSAGE AND INFANTS

In order to appreciate the scientific studies about infant massage, we need to look at what was going on before the national consumer movement in the 1960s and 1970s. Prior to this era, the medical standard practice whisked babies off to the nursery immediately after birth to be monitored by nurses and physicians. This isolation of the newborn left mothers and fathers out of the events in the lives of their babies usually until the day of discharge, which was several days after the birth event. In the 1960s and 1970s several events took place that caused the medical profession to reexamine this practice.

First, was the patients' rights movement that proclaimed patients had the right to have some input and control over what medical interventions were carried out. And second, was a major scientific piece of work done by Drs. Klaus and Kennell and published in a book, called *Mother—Infant Bonding*. Their work identified that touch was crucial for the development of the normal parent-infant attachment, and that there is a critical time window for this attachment to begin that includes the first hours and days after the birth.

This study on mother-infant bonding was revolutionary in that it changed how obstetricians conducted labor and how pediatricians managed their newborn patients. Family centered maternity wards sprung up in every hospital. Rooming-in was made available to mothers. Fathers were no longer excluded from the labor room or the delivery room. And many women elected to deliver their babies at home.

The family who did not benefit from all these changes was the family who was unfortunate enough to give birth to an infant before it was considered mature, or a preterm infant. Preterm infants are at risk for many life-threatening problems associated with prematurity. Immediately after birth, the "preemie" baby is taken away to the Neonatal Intensive Care Unit where the ultimate in medical technology is applied. It was thought the less these babies were handled or exposed to germs from adults, the less they risked catching illnesses when the babies were poorly equipped to survive, much less, fight infections.

As child development studies evolved dealing with preterm infants, it was found that their was poor parent-infant bonding in the family triad (mother, baby, father). It was felt that this resulted from parents not being allowed extended time in the NICU to interact with their preterm babies.

Innovative programs began to invite the parents and even grandparents into the NICU settings with no dire effects. Recognizing the importance and power of touch, NICU staffs began to encourage parents to touch and hold their infants. Mothers were allowed to nurse their babies. They were encouraged to pump their breasts and bring in the milk for feeding.

Many studies looked at physiological responses of the babies associated with parental and caregiver touch. They found there were no adverse effects associated with parent touching and many positive effects including parent satisfaction.

However, until the work of Tiffany Fields, Ph.D., in the '80s there were no published studies looking at the effects of a massage regimen in addition to the parental-caregiver touch in infants, preterm or otherwise. Her study results were positive, showing increased weight gain and neurological maturation in the preterm infants exposed to massage.

Dr. Field describes the infant massage techniques on the premature babies as Swedish massage that included "stroking from the thigh to the foot and back to the thigh," and "stroking from the shoulder to the wrist and back to the shoulder." The technique did not include any squeezing or twisting. The studies she performed using light stroking demonstrated that the infants had a dislike for this type of touch and gained less weight and demonstrated less neurological development.

INFANT MASSAGE TECHNIQUES

I propose that massage therapists examine the use of the Indian technique of infant massage described as squeezing, twisting, and stroking from the shoulder to the hand, and from the thigh to the foot pushing blood against the natural flow of the blood current.

My suggestion for this examination is twofold:
1. Anatomy and physiology of the venous system
2. Promotion of professional integrity

ANATOMY AND PHYSIOLOGY OF THE VEINS IN THE INFANT AND ADULT

Veins are the blood vessels that carry blood back to the heart from all parts of the body. Because the veins in the legs and arms have to conduct the flow of blood against the pull of gravity, they have valves. These valves serve to prevent backward flow or reflux of blood on its way back to the heart.

The valves are semilunar in shape and look like little horseshoe sacs attached to the walls of the veins. There are almost always two sacs opposite each other, in some locations three sacs, and occasionally one sac. They lie close to the wall of the vein as long as the current of blood is flowing naturally. With any back flow of blood due to a barrier (tourniquet for example) the valves fill with blood, expand, and swell. Their opposed edges meet and the backward flow of blood is interrupted. (See Figure 24.)

According to *Gray's Anatomy,* Henry S. Gray, Lea & Febiger, and *Nelson's Textbook Of Pediatrics,* Richard Behrman, M.D., W. B. Saunders Co., there is no difference in the venous system of an adult and an infant. The infant's system is smaller and more delicate.

How does the presence of valves in the veins of the extremities impact on massage technique?

Swedish massage refers to and acknowledges development by Peter Henrik Ling, a Swedish gymnastics instructor who synthesized Greek, Chinese, Egyptian, and Roman techniques into massage. During Ling's lifetime, physicians around the world looked to Swedish medical schools for information on massage. Today his techniques are taught in schools of massage across the United States.

Ling's Swedish massage techniques take into account the anatomy and physiology of the venous system and the role of the valves located in veins in the limbs. He advocates that massage of the limbs other than light stroking always be done with stroking, squeezing, or twisting towards the heart, not away from the heart. This type of stroking facilitates the blood flow current. Stroking away from the heart can act as a barrier creating a back flow that has the potential to damage the valves in the veins. Damaged valves can result in varicose veins.

It appeals to reason if this type of stroking is contraindicated in the adult, it is contraindicated in the infant and has the potential to damage delicate valves in the venous system of the limbs of an infant. The Indian version of infant massage as practiced by the women in India on their babies and taught in this country—squeezing, twisting, and stroking of the extremities away from the heart, against the natural flow of the bloodstream—should be adapted to squeeze, twist, and stroke toward the heart, following the flow of the blood from hand to shoulder and foot to thigh.

In 1993 at a grant-writing seminar sponsored by the National Institute of Health, I had the opportunity to meet several physicians educated in India who practiced Aryvedic medicine here in the United States. They were eager to answer my questions about why Indian mothers performing massage on their babies stroke away from the heart instead of toward the heart. In order to understand why this technique is used, they explained that Aryvedic medicine, among other things, deals with energy fields. The Indian mother performs this technique at the beginning of the massage to rid the infant of negative energy.

Promotion of professional integrity is of particular importance. Members of the massage profession write the rules and decide what is appropriate, therapeutic, and safe especially for massage used on infants.

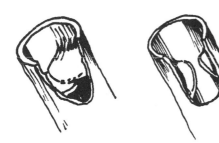

Figure 24

Valves in veins.

Is Infant massage a service the massage therapist should offer?

Utilizing one of the how-to books listed above, the massage therapist should have no misgivings about adding infant massage to their list of skills. The how-to books are written to teach parents how to massage their babies. The techniques are easy to learn and to teach. It is a simple matter to modify the direction of the squeezing, twisting, and stroking of the extremities of the infant to follow the natural direction of the current of blood.

Massage therapists are the experts on massage. This does not mean that every massage therapist is a teacher. Teaching massage rather than performing massage requires different skills. Those massage therapists who feel some intimidation sitting in comfortable, familiar surroundings with their clients, teaching them how to massage their infants certainly should seek help with teaching techniques from such organizations as the International Association of Infant Massage Instructors or programs offered at the massage schools.

How do you market infant massage instruction?

There is no marketing data available about how willing or financially able new young parents are to purchase the services of an infant massage instructor. Empirical data garnered from offering infant massage instruction for five years at a massage facility in central Florida show classes made available for free were well received. Classes advertised for pay were not so popular.

Infant massage as part of a prenatal, doula, postpartum package is much better received. Placing the infant massage service within the prenatal massage as free seems to work well and can be a marketing give-away. Infant massage classes can be a creative shower gift, for a fee.

Use your knowledge and skills of infant massage and approach the nursing personnel at the local hospital with a nursery. Volunteer to teach nurses, parents, and grandparents the techniques and benefits of infant massage.

Use the work done by Dr. Field and ask to work with any cocaine babies or HIV-exposed babies. Offer to teach the parents of the "at-risk" babies. Dr. Field's research shows that the parents, as well as the infants, benefit from infant massage. (A list of some of studies done by Dr. Field appears in the Appendix at the end of this book.)

Visit the offices of the local pediatricians. Offer to teach their staff about infant massage. Pediatricians are busy people and the massage therapist who demonstrates respect for their busy schedule will find a friendly reception.

A technique that has worked well for me is a brief visit during office hours. Purchase a couple of carnations wrapped with greenery from a florist. Ask the receptionist to give the flowers along with your card and a flier or one-page description about infant massage. Ask for a couple of minutes to introduce yourself, or ask for a more convenient time that you could return. Ask for permission to leave your card or advertisement fliers in the waiting room. Ask your clients to give your infant massage material to their pediatrician.

When do you start infant massage classes?

You should prepare your parents for the class in the prenatal period by asking them to purchase and read whatever infant massage how-to book you recommend before the birth of the baby. With their homework out of the way before the baby is born, both parents can attend the infant massage class, making it a fun and relaxed time for all parties. Most of the books recommend starting infant massage no sooner than three weeks of age. Extrapolating from the work of Dr. Field, if massage of premature babies is healthy and desirable, infant massage on a normal infant is safe at any age.

Chapter Eight

MARKETING/RESEARCH/RECORD KEEPING

MARKETING

Marketing massage for pregnancy is basically the same as any other marketing activity. However, it is important to understand how to tap medical professionals to work with you and to support your contribution to a healthy mother and baby. Preparing yourself to help your client explore reimbursement from health insurance is also a plus for you. The components of marketing for massage include:

1. Community recognition. Community recognition begins with advertisements in local newspapers. These can be ads in the classified section, which are fairly inexpensive, or display ads. The smaller newspapers are an excellent place to get free advertising through news releases. A news release can be about anything related to massage and your activities as a therapist. If you attend a seminar or a convention, write up a short description of where it was held, how many people attended, the theme, or a sentence or two of what you found interesting. Send it or deliver it in person to the editor along with a photo of you at the meeting or you at work at your facility.

   The larger newspapers usually have a policy of not using the above type of news releases, but they have regular columns for community announcements and will print information about new services or educational classes or meetings in which you can mention yourself or your business. Sponsor a speaker. Announce it in the papers. Distribute advertising fliers about the event. Even if only a few people show up, you get many dollars worth of free advertisement.

Get permission to leave advertisement fliers at physicians' and chiropractors' offices, beauty salons, colleges, etc. Volunteer for presentations about massage at civic meetings. Take your massage chair with you. Nothing works better than a hands-on demonstration. Get to know the childbirth educators in the community.

2. Using word of mouth. This is the work of the satisfied customer. Do not be bashful. Ask them to spread the word if they like what you do for them. Furnish your clients with fliers about prenatal massage. Ask them to tell their physician, midwife, and childbirth teacher. Ask for testimonial letters about their experience with massage and how they felt it impacted on their labor and birth. Make a booklet of these testimonials for your waiting room. Make extra copies of the booklet to leave with your cards at other waiting rooms.

3. Gatekeepers and influence factors. Understanding and use of influence factors surrounding massage of pregnant women and how to get past the gatekeepers to health care insurance money is important. Many therapists receive nonpregnant client referrals from physicians especially for pain control or to promote healing from injuries.

Pregnancy is a normal physiologic state, not an illness. It is marked by many physical adaptations beginning a few days after conception. What does a massage therapists need to know about pregnancy in order to ask the physician and the midwife to refer pregnant clients? Physiological adaptations of pregnancy.

The therapist who can discuss pregnancy in terms of physiology and the body's adaptation to pregnancy is in a position to influence midwives and physicians and thereby gain referrals.

Influence also refers to who controls the health care money. (See Table 2.) Until the health care system changes, your client's ability to pay for your services may be tied to her health care insurance program. Health care in the United States is a disease-driven system, not a preventive system, and your work with pregnant clients will be mainly preventive.

Table 2

MONEYTREE
"The Gatekeepers"

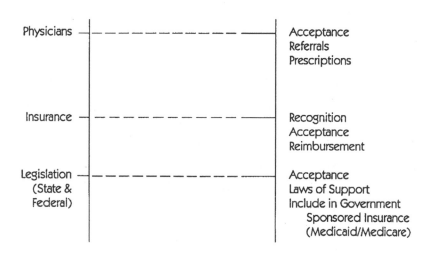

Physicians		Acceptance Referrals Prescriptions
Insurance		Recognition Acceptance Reimbursement

Legislation
(State &
Federal)
		Acceptance
		Laws of Support
		Include in Government
		    Sponsored Insurance
		    (Medicaid/Medicare)

Health Care in the USA is a Disease-Driven System
versus
A Preventive Care System

As you may already know, health insurance programs are regulated by gatekeepers. The power of the gatekeeper is established and supported by state and federal government legislation. A classic example of how this works is the way drugs are sold. Many prescription drugs that can only be obtained by paying money to see the physician (gatekeeper) are available over-the-counter in countries like Canada and Mexico.

Reimbursement from major medical insurance companies for massage in pregnancy is within the power of the physician. The physician decides and chooses the type of services needed to promote a healthy pregnancy—laboratory tests, sonograms, etc., and writes prescriptions or orders for these services. Laboratory tests and other measures, prescribed or ordered by the physician, are considered for payment by health insurance programs. When the physician writes a prescription for massage, many major medical insurance programs will pay some amount of the charge.

In order for you to tap into the "money tree," you must use the "influence tree." (See Table 3.) Your influence tree consists of your patient as your advocate. She is the customer of the physician, meaning she has the power to bring her insurance dollars or private dollars to her physician. She will have more clout than you in getting a prescription for massage from her medical provider.

Also, do not overlook the nurse-midwife or the nurse practitioner. In many states these practitioners are authorized to write prescriptions and may order services such as massage. Nurse-midwives are experts in normal pregnancy and work in a collaborative relationship with a physician. The nurse-midwife will probably be more open to massage in pregnancy since their area of expertise is the normal pregnancy. Their practice has an underlying philosophy of preventive and low-technology health care.

Table 3

Influence Tree

| Patient Advocate | Patient | Medical Doctor
Doctor of Osteopathy
Doctor of Chiropractor
Podiatrist
Certified Nurse Midwife
ObGyn Nurse Practitioner. | Prenatal
Postnatal
Infant
Massage | Rreferrals
and
Prescriptions |

Pricing Your Work

The following pricing formula used at New Image Wellness Center since 1990 has worked quite well. The regular advertised price for a one-hour massage is $60. Clients who choose to come for massage on a weekly basis get a price reduction to $150 per month. This equates to $30 per massage using a five-week month. The regular price for a series of Infant Massage classes is $75. Infant massage is hard to sell, so it is included as part of the prenatal massage package as free.

Table 4 shows the pricing of a massage package based on the first massage given at 14-weeks gestation through 40-weeks gestation, equaling a fee of $780. Six weeks of weekly massage in the postpartum period equals $180. During the postpartum period a weekly session (for four weeks with both parents) for teaching infant massage, which is free, gives a grand total of $960.

Table 4

Pricing Your Work

Regular price for a one hour massage at New Image Wellness Center is $60. Lowest rate is
a monthly price of $150. This equates to $30 per massage if you use a five week month.

Regular price for five infant massage sessions $75. Infant massage is very hard to sell, so it
is a give-away to our prenatal clients.

Suggested

14 Weeks	thru	40 Weeks	=	26 wk x $30	=	$780
Postpartum			=	6 wk x $30	=	$180
Infant massage Instru			=	5 wk		Free
				Total	·	$960

Regular charges should reflect professional service charges. Cannot use one price for
cash and a higher price for insurance purposes.

Comparison of Fees

Hours spent with client prenatally by caregivers:

Physician	2 to 3 Hrs	Fee	$2500 - $3000
Midwife	21 Hrs		$1100 - $1800
LMT	37 Hrs		$ 960

How does one justify the price of their services? The price
can be based on fees charged by other therapists, which is com-
petition driven. Another way to look at pricing is the amount of
time or hours spent with the client. Table 4 shows hours spent
with the pregnant woman and the average fee in central Florida
ranked by physician, midwife, and massage therapist. The physician spends the least amount of time with the pregnant client
and charges the most money. The midwife spends many more
hours with the client and usually charges less than the physician. The massage therapist spends the most number of hours
with the pregnant client—massage begins at 14-weeks gestation—more hours than the physician or the midwife and charges
the least amount of money.

Another way to look at the money equation is savings. If the work of the massage therapist reduces even one episode of premature labor, the savings of medical costs to stop one episode of premature labor will more than pay for the entire course of massage during the pregnancy. The charge for massage service is a mere drop in the bucket when medical intervention fails to prevent the birth of a premature baby. This event can cost thousands of dollars in hospital and physician charges. Tax dollars needed for care and education over the lifetime of a damaged child adds much more to the cost resulting from premature birth. The study by Dr. Tiffany Field of massage of premature infants resulted in fewer hospitalization days for the "preemies" resulting in savings of health care dollars of approximately $3,000 per baby.

The medical community and insurance companies are very much aware of potential expenses. Documentation through research of the benefits of massage in pregnancy that saves money will send insurance companies and physicians to your door looking for savings in health care dollars.

RESEARCH

What is research? *Webster's New Collegiate Dictionary* states, "research means to search again or to examine." More specifically, in scientific terms, it is a diligent, systematic inquiry or investigation to validate old knowledge or to generate new knowledge. A systematic and diligent inquiry requires planning, organization, and persistence.

Doing research sounds intimidating but can be very simple. Ask what needs to be known? How can it be measured? How can other elements or events of the world be prevented from interfering with the measurement? What meaning can be extracted from the measurements? These activities, questioning, planning, observing, analyzing, and explaining, are the "elements of research."

Why Is Research Necessary?

Research generates a scientific body of knowledge and theories that have been tested. In many instances, the knowledge and theories of massage therapy are based on ancient knowledge and techniques, many of them are not generated in our western culture. However, there exists multitudes of empirical data associated with massage in the western culture. Empirical data refers to the world as we experience it through our senses. Another way to describe empirical data is the stories your clients tell you about their experiences and the stories massage therapists tell each other about their experiences. In the scientific arena, empirical data is used to generate ideas for further questioning, observing, measuring, explaining, and analyzing—research.

The development of a scientific basis for the practice of massage through research is essential to moving the profession of massage into mainstream health care and routine obstetric care. Research is essential to the development of the profession of massage.

Definition Of A Profession

The definition of a profession includes several components. There exists a body of scientifically proven knowledge. The members of the profession have control of what they do within the practice of applying that knowledge. The members write the rules, and have the autonomy to make decisions and define what its practitioners will and will not do. No other group of people can decide the limits of what is appropriate for a member to practice.

Massage and touch therapy is a way of seeing people and teaching them to see and experience themselves and their world that is really different from other sciences. Massage tends toward a holistic view of humans, the person is greater than the sum of her parts. When you use the discipline of other professions to define massage, the focus shifts away from the touch/ massage orientation.

There are hundreds of massage therapists in practice who have the skills to do research. The bachelor, master, or doctorate degrees that provide the skills for formal scientific study are acquired within colleges and universities. However, the profession of massage attracts and is embraced by people who already have these degrees. There are hundreds of massage therapists in practice today who have the skills to do research.

Members of a "profession" identify their particular areas of concern and conduct research of these areas. They develop a body of scientific knowledge. Developing and testing of theories through research enhances the accountability of the profession. A solid research base will provide evidence of the massage actions necessary to promote good health and prevent disease. Outcomes can be accurately predicted as a result of massage and touch intervention.

The use of research will make the massage therapist more credible as an expert in the promotion and maintenance of healing and good health. Credibility, power, control, and accountability are related to the attainment of a true professional status and the platform for moving into mainstream health care.

Who Can Do Research?

Everyone. You have already studied and developed your theories of healing techniques. You are practicing them. You have overwhelming empirical data. Each time a new or old client comes to you, you make or modify a plan. A formal record of this plan may not be completed, but the process takes place. The therapist is engaged in observing each time a client gets off the massage table.

What Techniques Are You Already Doing That You Want To Measure?

Develop the measurement tool, compile, and analyze the information gained from the tool, and share this information with other members of your profession.

Those of you who like to read, go to the library and review what literature is already published on a single subject. Write a review of the available information and send the review to different journals for publication. Review of the literature is research and is a valuable contribution to the profession of massage.

Why Talk About Research In A Book About Massage For Pregnancy?

The massage profession has a window of opportunity to become part of routine obstetrical care. Consider what it would mean to your practice and your profession to be included for weekly therapeutic massage of pregnant women in the city where you practice. Consider what it would mean to your profession if the health care system saw massage as a way to save health care dollars.

Ask your local, state, and national professional organizations to set up a specialty for massage and pregnancy. Define what a massage therapist needs to know to practice this specialty. Encourage the schools to teach this specialty. Use the members of your profession who are interested in massage during pregnancy to compile their outcomes. As a group of professionals safely practicing the specialty of prenatal massage, measuring the outcomes of your client's pregnancies will build an indisputable body of knowledge. Outcomes should include:

- Number of clients in your caseload.
- Premature labor corrected by medical intervention.
- Number of premature labor episodes.
- Number of premature births.
- Length of labors.
- Number of deliveries by cesarean.
- Weight of baby at birth.
- Number of days hospitalized due to prematurity or other problem.
- Costs of hospital care resulting from premature birth.

Be sure to include other complications at birth. To be statistically significant, data from large numbers of pregnant women who received massage during pregnancy will be necessary to be convincing. This is especially true since the massage profession is not promoted by universities and major institutions such as the National Institute of Health with money to spend on research and reputations established to warrant acceptance.

RECORD KEEPING

The massage therapist practicing today is keeping records, if nothing else, financial records for tax purposes. Most practitioners take some type of written history, usually a checklist filled out by the client, with a simple figure of the human body for indicating painful areas.

Whatever type of client records currently in use, simple or elaborate, there are some simple standard documentations that need to be done concerning massage of the pregnant client. Most insurance companies will require some type of information on those clients who receive reimbursement for massage services. Establishment and maintenance of a system of recording client treatment information is an important tool for documentation of your techniques. It should include positioning on the table and progress. The documentation also serves as a tool to provide proof that massage treatment is necessary and curative—research documentation.

Figure 25 is a sample form that can be copied for use. Figure 26 is a simple form to be used after each massage. It contains a checklist of assessment before each massage session and has space for utilizing the SOAP charting system. These forms may be copied for use. Preparing SOAP notes is an easy, simple, and consistent method of documenting massage work.

Figure 25

Previous Pregnancies							
No.	Year	Place Delivered	Vaginal or C-Section	Hours of Labor	Weight of Baby	Complications Mother	Child

Figure 26

Date					
Number Weeks Gestation					
Edema					
Homan's Sign					
Table Position Used					
L Lateral Tilt					
L Lateral Lie					
R Lateral Lie					

SOAP is an acronym for Subjective, Objective, Assessment, Plan. Subjective refers to what the patient says about her condition. Objective refers to what you can see or measure with whatever tools you may be using to assess the condition of the client. For example, the client may say she has pain in her low back. This is subjective. When you examine her back and discover either muscle spasm or no evidence of muscle spasm, this is objective information.

Assessment is a summary of what she has told you and what you have been able to find on exam and/or measure. The important rule applied to assessment is information about the assessment appears either in what the client told you or what was found on exam and/or measured. There may be more than one assessment. Assessment in the above example would be low back pain secondary to muscle spasm. Plan is what you as her health caregiver, within the scope of your education, plan to do about the assessment of muscle spasm in the low back.

Example No 1: (No problem)

S)   Feels well, no complaints. States midwife says pregnancy is fine.

O)   Normal gait, no edema, Homan's negative.

A)   24-weeks pregnant, no problems found.

P)   Routine massage utilizing left tilt, L and R lateral lie.

Example No 2: (Problem)

S)   States she has pain in her low back for two days. Was afraid to take any medications. Used heating pad.

O)   1. Moderate muscle spasm located in the right lumbar area.

       2. Tenderness from top of sacrum to mid area maxi mus gluteus.

       3. Homan's sign negative.

A)   1. Low back pain secondary to muscle spasm on right.

       2. 25-weeks pregnant, no complaints of problems with pregnancy.

P)   1. Review good body mechanics while lifting.

       2. Suggest hot water bottle, stop heating pad to avoid danger of too much heat.

       3. Demonstrate how to arise from a lying position to protect back.

       4. Therapeutic massage with extra attention to area of muscle spasm using left lateral tilt and right and left lateral lie.

       5. Advised to consult midwife about pain medication if needed.

An excellent resource book written specifically for massage therapists on SOAP charting is *Hands Heal: Documentation For Massage Therapy, A Guide To SOAP Charting,* by Diana L. Thompson, LMP. The address for ordering this book is:

Healing Arts Studio
916 N.E. 64th
Seattle, WA 98115

Chapter Nine

HANDS-ON AND HOW-TO

Massage During Pregnancy is a how-to text for practicing massage therapists, individuals seeking advanced study in the specialty field of prenatal massage, students enrolled in schools of massage, and other students of massage. Your skills include basic massage techniques. Throughout the preceding pages the role of the massage therapist in pregnancy has been discussed.

When To Begin Massaging The Pregnant Client And Why

Anywhere from ten to fifteen percent of all diagnosed pregnancies will end in spontaneous miscarriage before the end of the first trimester (13 weeks). If you include those pregnancies that result in miscarriage in the first several weeks before the diagnosis of pregnancy has been officially made, the rate rises to more than forty percent.

Spontaneous miscarriages before 8-weeks gestation are usually a result of an abnormal development of the egg, the embryo, or the placenta. Spontaneous miscarriages after 8-weeks gestation are usually caused by some genetic mutation of the fetus or illness or infection in the mother. Once the mother carries her pregnancy past the first trimester, the chances of having a successful pregnancy increase tremendously.

There is no known connection between massage and early pregnancy loss. Massage does not cause spontaneous miscarriage. However, pregnant families who experience spontaneous miscarriage will have grief and guilt associated with the loss. It is an easy mental exercise to shift blame to the doctor or the midwife for not performing adequate care, or to the massage therapist who touched in a new and different manner.

For this reason NEW massage clients who are pregnant should have completed the first trimester (13-weeks gestation). By not accepting new clients in the first trimester, the massage therapist completely avoids the possibility of a client associating miscarriage with any technique or modality performed by the therapist during this period. Established female clients of childbearing age present the possibility of massage before pregnancy is diagnosed. With this type of client, continuation of massage is acceptable. The therapist will have already established a bond and a trust level that precludes projections of blame or guilt in the event of spontaneous miscarriage. With established clients the massage therapist is usually viewed as part of the client's support network while grieving the loss.

Protect your reputation and your integrity. Establish the above policy and stick to it.

MASSAGE CONTRAINDICATIONS

There are few absolute contraindications for performing massage on the pregnant client. However, the ones that exist are important.

1. In the presence of a positive Homan's sign massage should be postponed and your client instructed to immediately contact her medical provider.

2. Massage of the breasts in a pregnant woman should not be done because stimulation of the breasts and nipples can cause her to have contractions.

3. Do not place your pregnant client in the supine position for massage if she is past 13-weeks (3-months) gestation.

4. Massage should not be performed on the client with a problem of high blood pressure.

5. Massage should not be done in the presence of abnormal edema until this condition can be evaluated by her medical provider. Abnormal edema can indicate a problem with elevated blood pressure.

6. Heat in the form of hot packs or heliotherapy should not be applied to the abdomen or flank.

7. Medical problems that contraindicate massage in the non-pregnant client apply to the pregnant client.

POSITIONING OF THE PREGNANT CLIENT ON THE MASSAGE TABLE

Traditionally, the supine and prone positions are used for performing massage. The supine position in the pregnant woman is contraindicated after 13-weeks gestation in order to avoid Supine Hypotensive Syndrome.

Alternatives to the supine position is the "left lateral tilt" or "Fowler's position." Alternatives to the prone position are the "left lateral lie" and the "right lateral lie."

Left Lateral Tilt

This is a position that can be safely used at any month of the pregnancy. The left lateral tilt consists of placing a rolled blanket or wedge under the right side of the woman tilting her toward the left. The blanket should be large enough to raise her right shoulder, ribs, and flank approximately 15 degrees. The support of the blanket or wedge should reach from her right shoulder down as far as the top of the iliac crest. In this position the weight of the uterus falls toward the left flank and abdominal wall avoiding pressure on the aorta and the vena cava—

preventing supine hypotensive syndrome. (See Figure 27.) The sequelae of Supine Hypotensive Syndrome is discussed in Chapter One.

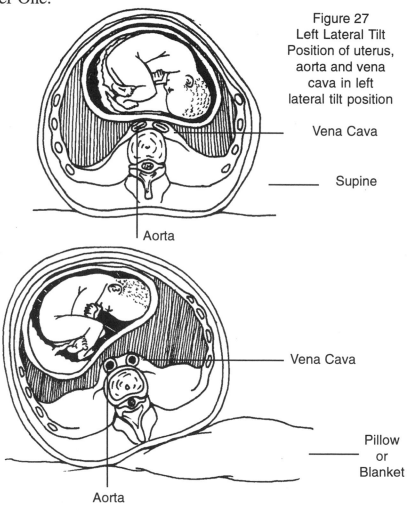

Figure 27
Left Lateral Tilt
Position of uterus,
aorta and vena
cava in left
lateral tilt position

Vena Cava

Supine

Aorta

Vena Cava

Pillow
or
Blanket

Aorta

This position allows the therapist easy access to work on the head, face, neck, and arms while standing or seated at the head of the table. Massage of the arms and shoulders, including any range of motion of the arms and shoulders can be done from either side of the table with the client in left lateral tilt. Massage of the abdomen, anterior portion of the legs and the feet can also be completed with the client in this position.

Fowler's Position

This position was named by George R. Fowler, M.D., an American surgeon who died in the early 1900s. Fowler's position places the pregnant woman in a semi-sitting position and is described as placing the client's head 18 to 20 inches above the level of the table. This position prevents the uterus from falling back upon the pelvic rim, pressing on the aorta and vena cava. (See Figure 28.)

Fowler's position allows for good access to the client from either side of the table and can be used for massage of the face, head, shoulders, arms, hands, abdomen, legs, and feet. In the Fowler's position, you may want to place a soft narrow pillow under your client's knees, using your client's comfort level to guide you. This position will prevent Supine Hypotensive Syndrome at any month of the pregnancy. Your clients may find this position more comfortable in the last couple months of the pregnancy rather than left lateral tilt. The Fowler position works better if the massage table breaks to support the head and shoulders. (See Figure 29.) A single wedge can be used but it is necessary to anchor it in position to keep it from sliding off the end of the table. Pillows that raise the head and shoulders to the recommended height also require some type of anchor. A sheet spread over the wedge or pillows with the client reclining and sitting on top of the sheet can be used as a stabilizer. Placing the head of the table against a wall can also be a stabilizer for a wedge or pillows.

Figure 28

Fowlers position using a wedge

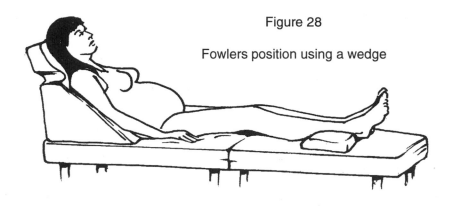

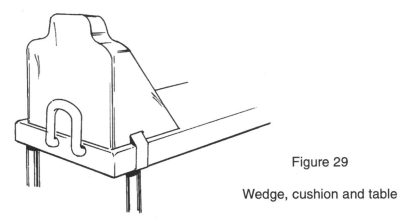

Figure 29

Wedge, cushion and table

(Available from
Jerry Curwin
New Image Wellness
Center
146 18th St. NW
Ruskin, FL 33570)

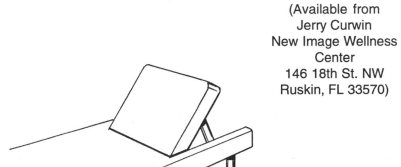

Left Lateral Lie

Left lateral lie is the very best position for the pregnant client while performing massage. Optimum circulation is accomplished with the pregnant woman in the left lateral lie position. While lying in this position she will have greater blood return to the heart because the weight of the body is off the aorta and the vena cava. The weight of the uterus will be on the left lateral wall of the abdomen and not pressing on any vital organs. Lying in this position also lowers the blood pressure.

Pillows from any department store or any of the commercial massage pillows may be used for support of the client when lying on her side. Use a firm pillow that supports the head at a comfortable level for the client. A firm pillow for the resting of the right thigh, knee, and leg is necessary. This pillow should be long enough to support the right leg from the knee past the ankle. This support should be high enough and firm enough to keep her shoulders, back, and hips aligned in a straight position avoiding any twisting of the spine. The left leg is extended in alignment with the back. Make sure there is no unnecessary pulling or pressure on the shoulders or the hips from the weight of the arms and legs. (See Figure 30.)

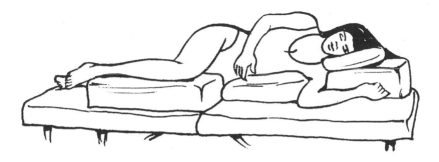

Figure 30

Left Lateral Lie

Small soft pillows can be used to tuck in front to support the abdomen and the uterus. A small pillow under the left ankle lying on the table will offer comfort and support. Some women may find it comfortable to have a small soft pillow placed at the back above the hips for support.

When placing your client in the left or right lateral lie position, guide her in sliding her back close to the edge of the table allowing more room for her arms and legs. This also provides you with complete access to the back for your massage work.

This allows for long smooth strokes from the top of the shoulders to the buttocks area. And, massage of the right buttocks, the right leg, and the medial aspect of the left leg can easily be done.

Right Lateral Lie

The right lateral lie position is an excellent position to place the client in to complete the massage. Massage of the left buttocks area, left leg and foot, and the medial aspect of the right leg can be done with ease. The positioning is the same as left lateral lie just reversed with the same type of pillow support. (See Figure 31.)

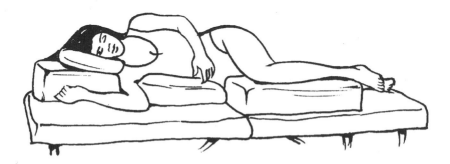

Figure 31

Right Lateral Lie

Prone Position

The prone position is contraindicated when massaging the pregnant client. The weight of the torso pushing down on the abdomen makes it very uncomfortable for the pregnant woman to lie on her abdomen. The individual who may be able to tolerate this position, comfort-wise, will have some impairment of blood flow.

The pressure of the weight of the uterus pushing upwards and gravity's downward pull can impair blood flow to the uterus. Any pressure applied to the back or buttocks by the therapist with the woman in the prone position can also increase the pressure on the great vessels.

Play it safe, delete the prone position from your massage technique of the pregnant client along with the supine position.

MASSAGE STROKES AND MODALITIES

In sixteen years of working with pregnant women as a nurse and a nurse-midwife, nine years operating a wellness center and massage establishment, knowledge of the anatomical and physiological changes associated with pregnancy, I know of no massage techniques taught in the traditional schools of massage that could be harmful to the pregnant woman. I know of no modalities practiced in traditional massage that could be harmful.

Most of the books on acupressure, such as reflexology and shiatsu, caution that stimulation of certain anatomical points and energy meridians will create labor. Location of these anatomical points are identified around the ankles, at the knees and LI4. (See Figure 20.) Except for the studies done by Dundee, et al. and Elizabeth Hyde, CNM, who examined acupressure therapy for the reduction of morning sickness, there are no quantitative data available dealing with acupressure and any aspect of pregnancy.

The following techniques are considered appropriate for use on the pregnant client:

- Swedish
- Neuromuscular therapy
- Craniosacral
- Polarity
- Touch for Health
- Muscle testing
- Reflexology—avoid anatomical points in (See Figure 20.)
- Shiatsu—avoid anatomical points in (See Figure 20.)
- Therapeutic Touch
- Most mind/body therapies

What About Perineal Massage?

From time to time, I have pregnant clients in my midwifery practice ask me about perineal massage. I was first introduced to perineal massage in 1979 while working at the Family Birthing Center of Providence Hospital, Southfield, Michigan. At the time, there was a strong underground lay-midwife movement in the Detroit area doing many home deliveries. Within the community of patients that delivered at the birthing center, perineal massage carried out by the woman's partner was popular.

Varney in her book *Midwifery* states that midwives who are "hands-on advocates" feel there are some advantages to manually stretching the perineum during the pushing stage of labor. In discussing several techniques for stretching the perineum during the pushing stage, she mentions perineal massage indicating it is used to promote perineal relaxation. She warns that if perineal massage is done "care should be taken that the use of oil not enter the perineum so there is no chance of its getting in the baby's mouth or respiratory tract."

My experience in midwifery practice has been that perineal massage during the pregnancy or during the labor does not appear to make any difference in whether or not the woman has lacerations at the time of the birth. Whether or not the woman suffers a perineal laceration depends on the skill of the person delivering the baby—physician or midwife. There is no data that shows that it shortens the pushing stage of labor.

Perineal massage carried out by a licensed massage therapist is contraindicated for no other reason than "touching the genitalia" is not within the scope of legitimate massage. Professional massage has struggled to move away from the "massage parlor" image. Massaging or advocating massage of the perineal area is not appropriate for the massage therapist.

Appendix 1

READING LIST FOR THE MASSAGE THERAPIST LABOR SUPPORT DOULA

Haire, Doris. THE CULTURAL WARPING OF CHILD-BIRTH. ICEA News Special Report. Seattle, Washington, ICEA Supply Center, 1972.

Jimenez, Sherry Lynn Mims. THE PREGNANT WOMAN'S COMFORT GUIDE, Prentice Hall, Inc., Englewood Cliffs, N.J. 1983.

Krieger, Delores. THE THERAPEUTIC TOUCH, Prentice Hall, Englewood Cliffs, N.J.1979.

Mitford, Jessica. THE AMERICAN WAY OF BIRTH, Penguin Books, USA, New York, 1992.

Peterson, Gayle, BIRTHING NORMALLY: A PERSONAL APPROACH TO CHILDBIRTH. Mindbody Press, Berkeley, CA.

Peterson, Gayle, Mehl, Lewis. PREGNANCY AS HEALING, Volume I and the chapter titled "Holistic Interventions During Labor" in Volume II. Mindbody Press, Berkeley, CA.

Perez, Paulina, Snedeker, Cheryl, SPECIAL WOMEN, THE ROLE OF THE PROFESSIONAL LABOR ASSISTANT, Pennypress, Seattle, WA, 1990.

Varney, Helen. NURSE-MIDWIFERY, Second Edition, Blackwell Scientific Publications, Boston. 1987.

Appendix 2

INFANT MASSAGE STUDIES

1. Field, Tiffany M., Ph.D., "Supplemental stimulation of preterm infants." *Early Human Development* 1980;4:301-14.

2. Field, T. M., et al., "Effects of tactile/kinesthetic stimulation on preterm neonates." *Pediatrics* 1986;77:654-8.

3. Field, T. M., et al., "Massage of preterm newborns to improve growth and development." *Pediatric Nurse* 1987;13:385-7.

4. Field, T. M., et al., "Tactile-kinesthetic stimulation effects on sympathetic and adrenocortical function in preterm infants." *Journal of Pediatrics*, 1991;3;119:434-40.

5. Field, T. M., et at., "Massage Reduces Anxiety in Child and Adolescent Psychiatric Patients." *Journal of the American Academy of Child Adolescent Psychiatry*, 31:1, Jan 1992:125-131.

6. Harrison, Woods, "Early Parental Touch and Preterm Infants." *JOGNN*, Jul/Aug 1991;20;4:299-306.

7. Werner, Conway, "Caregiver Contacts Experienced by Premature Infants in the Neonatal Intensive Care Unit." *Maternal-Child Nursing Journal*; 19; 1:21-41.

BIBLIOGRAPHY

Chapter One—The Anatomy and Physiology of Pregnancy

Bark, Joseph P., M.D., RETIN-A AND OTHER YOUTH MIRACLES, Prima Publishing & Communications, Rocklin, CA.

Bobak, Jensen, ESSENTIALS OF MATERNITY NURSING, Third Edition, Mosby Year-Book, Inc., St. Louis, MO. 1991.

Chapman, Cheryl, RN, LMT, "The Whole 9 Months, There's the Rub." Parenting Magazine, Nov. 1992:45.

Cunningham, MacDonald, Gant, WILLIAMS OBSTETRICS, Eighteenth Edition, Appleton & Lange, Norwalk, CT. 1989.

Miller, Keane, ENCYCLOPEDIA AND DICTIONARY OF MEDICINE AND NURSING, W. B. Saunders Company, Philadelphia, PA.

PHYSICIANS' DESK REFERENCE, 1994.

Varney, Helen, MIDWIFERY, Second Edition, Blackwell Scientific Publications, Boston, MA. 1987.

Walzer, Richard A., M.D., HEALTHY SKIN A Guide to Lifelong Skin Care, Consumer Reports Book, Consumers Union, Mount Vernon, NY. 1989.

Chapter Two—Discomforts of Pregnancy

Dundee, J. W., et al., "P6 Acupressure Reduces Morning Sickness." Journal Of The Royal Society Of Medicine, Aug. 1988:456-7.

Hyde, Elisabeth, CNM, MSN, "Acupressure Therapy for Morning Sickness." Journal Of Nurse-Midwifery, Vol. 34;4; Jul./Aug. 1989:171-78.

Jimenez, Sherry Lynn Mims, THE PREGNANT WOMAN'S COMFORT GUIDE, Prentice-Hall, Inc., Englewood Cliffs, NJ. 1983.

Varney, Helen, MIDWIFERY, Second Edition, Blackwell Scientific Publications, Boston, MA. 1987.

Chapter Three—Maternal Psychological Adjustment

Humenick, Sharron S., RN,Ph.D.,FAAN, "Your Labor Guide."
Lamaze Parents' Magazine, ASPO/Lamaze, 1994 Edition:58-64.

Peterson, Gayle, MSSW,LCSW and Mehl, Lewis, M.D.,Ph.D., PREG-
NANCY AS HEALING, A Holistic Philosophy for Prenatal
Care, Volumes I and II, Mindbody Press, Berkeley, CA. 1985.

Varney, Helen, MIDWIFERY, Second Edition, Blackwell Scientific
Publications, Boston, MA. 1987.

Chapter Four—Labor (Giving Birth)

Lieberman, Adrienne, EASING LABOR PAIN, Doubleday, Bantam
Dell Div, New York, NY.

Melzack, Ronald, M.D., "The McGill Pain Questionnaire: Major
Properties and Scoring Methods," Pain, 1; 1975:277-299.

Melzack, Ronald, M.D. and Bentley, K. C., M.D., "Relief of Dental
Pain by Ice Massage of Either Hand or the Contralateral Hand,"
Canadian Dental Assoc., 1983;49:257-260.

Melzack, Ronald, M.D. et al., "Relief of Dental Pain By Ice Massage
of the Hand," Canadian Medical Assoc., Jan. 26, 1980, 122:189-
191.

Melzack, R and Wall, P., "Pain Mechanisms: A New Theory," Science,
Nov. 19, 1965, Vol. 150, No. 3699:971-78.

Shapiro, Harriet Roberts, et al., THE LAMAZE READY-REFER-
ENCE GUIDE FOR LABOR & BIRTH, Shapira Kuba,
Rockville, M.D., 1990.

Simkin, Penny, PT, "Stress, Pain, and Catecholamines in Labor: Part 1.
A Review." Birth, 13:4, December 1986:227-33.

Stolte, Karen, RN, Ph.D., CNM, "A Comparison of Women's Expecta-
tions of Labor With the Actual Event." Birth, 14:2; June 1987:99-
103.

Torgerson, W. S., "What Objective Measures Are There for Evaluating
Pain?" The Journal Of Trauma, Sept. 1984, Vol. 24, No. 9
Supplement.

Waters, Bette, CNM, "Ice Massage for the Control of Labor Pain," a research paper presented at the University of Southern Queensland, Australia, as part of the Australian-American Nurses Exchange Program, 1992.

Yates, John, A PHYSICIAN'S GUIDE TO THERAPEUTIC MASSAGE: Its Physiological Effects and Their Application to Treatment." Massage Therapists' Association of British Columbia, Vancouver, BC, Canada, 1990.

Chapter Five—Massage Therapists as Doula

Hodnett, Ellen D. and Osborn, Richard W. "Effects of Continuous Intrapartum Professional Support on Childbirth Outcomes." Research in Nursing & Health, 12;1989:289-297.

Kennell, John, M.D. and Klaus, Marshall, M.D., et al., "Continuous Emotional Support During Labor in a US Hospital." Journal Of The American Medical Association, May 1, 1991; Vol. 265; No. 17:2197-2201.

Klaus, Marshall M.D. and Kennell, John M.D., et al., "Effects of Social Support During Parturition on Maternal and Infant Morbidity." British Medical Journal, Vol. 293; Sept. 6, 1986:585-87.

Letter, "Discover the Doula Conference," Midwifery Today, PO Box 2672, Eugene, OR, 97402; No.11, 1989:9

"Love's Labor Lessened." Newsweek; May 13, 1991:65.

Sosa, Roberto, M.D.; Kennell, John, M.D.; Klaus, Marshall, M.D., et al., "The Effect of a Supportive Companion on Perinatal Problems, Length of Labor, and Mother-Infant Interaction." The New England Journal Of Medicine, Vol. 303; No.11; Sept. 11, 1990:598-600.

Vincent, Kerry, Doula, "A Doula Mothers the Mother." Midwifery Today, PO Box 2672, Eugene, OR, 97402; No.9, 1989:17.

Vincent, Kerry, Doula, "The Birth and Growth of a Doula Service." Midwifery Today; No. 12,1989:16-17.

Chapter Six—The Postpartum Period

Cunnningham, MacDonald, Gant, WILLIAMS OBSTETRICS, 18th Edition, Appleton & Lange, Norwalk, CT. 1989.

Varney, Helen, MIDWIFERY, Second Edition, Blackwell Scientific Publications, Boston, MA. 1987.

Chapter Seven—Infant Massage

Auckett, Amelia, BABY MASSAGE, Hill of Content Publishing, Melbourne, Australia, 1989.

Behrman, Richard E., M.D., NELSON TEXTBOOK OF PEDIATRICS, 14th Edition, W. B. Saunders Co., Harcourt Brace Javanovich, Inc., Independence Square, Philadelphia, PA.

Field, Tiffany M., Ph.D., "Supplemental stimulation of preterm infants." Early Human Development 1980;4:301-14.

Field, T.M. et al., "Effects of tactile/kinesthetic stimulation on preterm neonates." Pediatrics 1986;77:654-8.

Field, T.M. et al., "Massage of preterm newborns to improve growth and development." Pediatric Nurse 1987;13;385-7.

Field, T.M., "The benefits of infant massage on growth and development." Pediatric Basics, Winter 95;71;8-12.

Field, T.M., et al., "Massage reduces anxiety in child and adolescent psychiatric patients." Journal Of American Academy Of Child And Adolescent Psychiatry, Jan. 1992;31:1:125-131.

Gray, Henry, FRS, GRAY'S ANATOMY, edited by Charles Mayo Goss, AB, M.D., Lea & Febiger, Philadelphia, PA. 1991.

Harrison, Woods, "Early Parental Touch an Preterm Infants." JOGNN, Jul./Aug. 1991;20;4:299-306.

Heinl, Tina, THE BABY MASSAGE BOOK, Coventure, Ltd, London, Boston, Mass. 1990.

Johnson & Johnson, Consumer Products, Inc., ADVANCES IN TOUCH, Pediatric Round Table: 14, edited by Gunzenhauser, Brazelton, Field. 1990.

Johnson & Johnson, Consumer Products, Inc., THE MANY FACETS OF TOUCH, Pediatric Round Table: 10, edited by Caldwell and Brazelton. 1984.

Leboyer, Frederick, M.D., LOVING HANDS, THE TRADITIONAL INDIAN ART OF BABY MASSAGE. Knops, a division of Random House, NY, 1976.

McClure, Vimala Schneider, INFANT MASSAGE A HANDBOOK FOR LOVING PARENTS, Bantam Books, New York, NY 1989.

Meyer, Tamara, HELP YOUR BABY BUILD A HEALTHY BODY, A New Exercise and Massage Program for the First Five Formative Years, Crown Publishers, Inc. New York, NY. 1984.

Tappan, Frances M., HEALING MASSAGE TECHNIQUES, Reston Publishing Company, Reston, VA. 1980.

Werner, Conway, "Caregiver Contacts Experienced by Premature Infants in the Neonatal Intensive Care Unit." Maternal Child Nursing Journal; 19;1:21-41.

Chapter Eight—Marketing/Research/Record Keeping

Burns, Nancy, and Grove, Susan, THE PRACTICE OF NURSING RESEARCH: CONDUCT, CRITIQUE AND UTILIZATION, W. B. Saunders, Philadelphia, PA, 1987.

Perrin, Kay, RN, MSN, Speech on marketing doula services at Prenatal Massage Seminar February, 1993, Ruskin, FL.

Spassof, Alex, LMT, Speech on marketing massage services at Prenatal Massage Seminar, February, 1993, Ruskin, FL.